T0202151

A History of Haematology

Oxford Medical Histories Series

This series of Oxford Medical Histories is designed to bring to a wide readership of clinical doctors and others from many backgrounds a short but comprehensive text setting out the essentials of differing areas of medicine. Volumes in this series are written by doctors and with doctors, in particular, in mind as the readership.

History describes the knowledge acquired over time by human beings. It is a form of storytelling, of organizing knowledge, of sorting and giving impetus to information. The study of medical history, just like the history of other human endeavours, enables us to analyse our knowledge of the past in order to plan our journey forward and hence try to limit repetition of our mistakes — a sort of planned process of Natural Selection, described as being in the tradition of one of the most famous of medical historians, William Osler. Medical history also encourages and trains us to use an academic approach to our studies which thereby should become more precise, more meaningful and more productive. Medical history should be enjoyable too, since that is a powerful stimulus to move forward, a fun thing to do both individually and in groups.

The inspiring book that led to this series introduced us to clinical neurology, genetics, and the history of those with muscular dystrophy. Alan and Marcia Emery explored *The History of a Genetic Disease*, now often styled Meryon's disease rather than Duchenne Muscular Dystrophy. The first to describe a disease process is not necessarily the owner of the eponym but the Emerys are helping put that right for their subject, Edward Meryon. The second book in the series, on radiology, took us on a journey round a world of images.

Thus future volumes in this series of Oxford Medical Histories will continue the journey through the history of our bodies, of their relationship to our environment, of the joyful and the sad situations that envelope us from our individual beginnings to our ends. We should travel towards other aspects of our humanity, always leaving us with more questions than answers since each new discovery leads to more questions, exponential sets of issues for us to study, further thoughts and attempts to solve the big questions that surround our existence. Medicine is about people and so is history; the study of the combination of the duo can be very powerful. What do you think?

Christopher Gardner-Thorpe, MD, FRCP, FACP

Series Advisor, Oxford Medical Histories

A History of Haematology

From Herodotus to HIV

Shaun R. McCann, Hon. FTCD

Professor Emeritus of Haematology and Academic Medicine,
St James' Hospital and Trinity College, Dublin,
Ireland

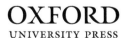
OXFORD
UNIVERSITY PRESS

UNIVERSITY PRESS

Great Clarendon Street, Oxford, OX2 6DP,
United Kingdom

Oxford University Press is a department of the University of Oxford.
It furthers the University's objective of excellence in research, scholarship,
and education by publishing worldwide. Oxford is a registered trade mark of
Oxford University Press in the UK and in certain other countries

Published in the United States of America by Oxford University Press
198 Madison Avenue, New York, NY 10016, United States of America

British Library Cataloguing in Publication Data
Data available

Library of Congress Control Number: 2015952899

ISBN 978–0–19–871760–7

Printed and bound by
CPI Group (UK) Ltd, Croydon, CR0 4YY

This book is dedicated to my wife, Brenda Moore-McCann, without whom it would never have seen the light of day. Her faith in me and her continuing support has been immeasurably helpful and I hope she enjoys reading the finished product.

'Patients want to know how much you care before they want to know how much you know'.

Professor Aidan Halligan (1957–2015)

Foreword

I like the dreams of the future better than the history of
the past

Thomas Jefferson, third president of the United States
of America (1743–1826), in a letter to John Adams,
dated 1 August 1816

When I was asked to submit a proposal for this book by Dr Christopher
Gardner-Thorpe, the series editor, I immediately agreed. I knew that Maxwell
M. Wintrobe had written two famous books about the history of haematology
in the 1980s, *Blood, Pure and Eloquent*, and *Hematology, The Blossoming of a
Science: A Story of Inspiration and Effort*. Both are excellent, with contributions
from many famous haematologists. Unfortunately, both books are now out of
print. Nonetheless, I have not repeated the ground covered by Wintrobe but
instead concentrated, with a few exceptions, on events in the last 25 years.

When I started as a 'Fellow' in haematology at the University of Minnesota
in the mid-1970s, haematology was still preoccupied with the physiology of
blood and concentrated mainly on benign blood diseases. There was effective
treatment for childhood acute lymphoblastic leukaemia and Hodgkin lymphoma, or Hodgkin's disease, as it was then called. Acute myeloid leukaemia,
although treated with combination chemotherapy, was almost universally
fatal, and non-Hodgkin lymphoma included a bewildering number of diseases
and classifications. Therapy consisted of a combination of radiation and chemotherapeutic agents and rarely, if ever, resulted in cure. Chronic myeloid leukaemia and multiple myeloma were depressing diseases to treat, with inevitable
mortality a few years after diagnosis. The term 'myelodysplasia' had not yet
been invented.

Widespread population migration had not yet taken place, with the exception
of the United States of America, and many red cell diseases such as sickle cell
disease and the thalassaemic syndromes were scarcely seen in European countries. Although treatment for haemophilia was available, support care for the
treatment of haematological malignancies was relatively underdeveloped. The
study of thrombosis, bleeding, and transfusion medicine had begun to separate
from 'general haematology', and this split became more obvious with the successful use of chemotherapy and haemopoietic stem cell transplantation.

The successful treatment of acute myeloid leukaemia and the advent of haematopoietic stem cell transplantation were associated with a surge in the development of support care, with improved venous access, treatment of infections, and platelet transfusions on demand. Haematopoietic stem cell transplantation was becoming available in most major haematology units by the mid-1980s.

Progress seemed to be in a linear direction until the epidemic of HIV/AIDS struck in the 1980s. There was a lack of interest among the general population and politicians, initially, as the disease appeared to be confined to prisoners and gay men. When it became clear that HIV/AIDS could affect the heterosexual population and that the disease was clearly spread by blood and blood product transfusion (before the virus was identified), the world sat up and reacted. Unfortunately, the reaction was not always helpful, and the disease became stigmatized. The transfusion services were severely stressed and, unfortunately, many people with haemophilia succumbed to HIV/AIDS.

At around the same time, genetics and molecular biology were beginning to undergo a revolution. In a strange way, the deaths of so many from HIV/AIDS provided a stimulus for the development of accurate testing of blood products for infectious agents, or antibodies to infectious agents. As a result, it is probably accurate to say that transfusion of blood and blood products has never been safer, from an infectious disease point of view, than they are today.

The development of automated cell counting and the widespread use of flow cytometry changed the diagnostic landscape for haematologists. The profusion of molecular techniques provided new investigations, new drugs, and a new understanding of the molecular basis of a number of both malignant and benign haematological diseases.

As always, changes in society occurred and these influenced the practice of medicine and haematology. Old 'paternalistic' attitudes began to change and patients gradually became more involved with their own disease/health. The training of medical students changed to accommodate this development and, at the same time, the number of women entering medical schools increased dramatically. Guidelines and new management styles of health services began to appear, augmented by European Union directives.

As outlined in the book, there were also changes in drug therapy. The major success story was the development of imatinib for the treatment of chronic myeloid leukaemia. This is a remarkable story and many of us know patients with chronic myeloid leukaemia who are alive and well 15 or more years from the time of their diagnosis. The use of monoclonal antibodies has been hugely beneficial, especially in the treatment of non-Hodgkin lymphoma.

On the downside, what has happened? Medical practice had undoubtedly become more bureaucratic, and doctors have, to some extent, lost the trust of the public. Doctors are losing the art of history taking and performing a thorough physical examination. There is an over-reliance on 'tests', and the costs of medicine to the state and to the individual are becoming unsustainable. In haematology, a careful examination of a well-made blood film is becoming a 'dying art', and morphological expertise has become compromised.

The culmination of the above is the idea of 'personalized' medicine. This phenomenon will certainly change the relationship between doctor and patient. Will doctors become less 'caring'? Will we create a cadre of the 'worried well'? Doctors must, of course, keep up with the latest developments but not at the cost of losing their ability to treat a patient humanely. The holistic management of patients, rather than the treatment of diseases, should be our goal. We must treat patients with respect and take adequate time to listen carefully to their story.

The outlook for patients with haematological diseases has never been better, but we as doctors, and not primarily scientists, must remember the words of the great Canadian physician and teacher, William Osler: 'The good physician treats the disease. The great physician treats the patient'. As a female colleague said to me recently, 'Perhaps a little bit of paternalism is not necessarily a bad thing!'

At a personal level, I am deeply indebted to my 'Chief of Hematology', Harry S. Jacob at the University of Minnesota, as he started me on a wonderful journey which culminated in my recent retirement as Professor of Haematology in St James' Hospital and Trinity College, Dublin.

Shaun R. McCann, Hon. FTCD
March 2015

Preface

I first met Dr Christopher Gardner-Thorpe, the editor of this series, at a dinner on the terrace of a mutual friend's house in Tuscany. The idea of a book on the 'History of Haematology' was consolidated over an excellent lunch in London sometime later and happily my proposal was, subsequently, accepted by Oxford University Press.

I have thoroughly enjoyed writing this book. I have always been fascinated by the phenomenon of people being 'written out of history' for whatever reason. Two examples are (1) that the Babylonians had 'cracked' the theorem of the square on the hypotenuse about 1800 years before Pythagoras, and (2) that the pulmonary circulation had been described hundreds of years before William Harvey's *De Motu Cordis*.

There are many intriguing questions to be answered but some of them relate to the changes that have taken place in man's imagination and thought processes over millennia. We have seen changes in attitudes to illness since the Greek idea that sickness was not caused by the gods but by natural phenomena. We have seen changes in writing styles and ideas and we have seen the replacement of the idea of beauty in art since the mid-1960s.

In medicine the ideas of Galen held sway for about 1500 years, and the idea of holistic medicine, attributed to Hippocrates, was intrinsic to medicine until recently. Hippocratic medicine was also distinguished by its interest in prognostication. The circle has been completed by the development of the concept of minimal or measurable residual disease and the stratification of treatment of patients with malignant haematological disorders and interventions based on 'probability'.

This book alludes to the ideas of the Greeks and how some Arabs have been written out of history. It examines the Enlightenment and the development of haematology since the invention of the microscope. The issues of war and its influence on medicine and haematology are also explored, as they have had huge implications for transfusion medicine and have contributed to the unravelling of stem cell biology.

The doctor/patient relationship has been a constant in Western medicine for thousands of years. Technological developments in imaging and the genetic and molecular revolutions have undoubtedly had a great impact on haematology, and many patients have benefited from these developments. The book outlines these developments but also asks some questions.

While not wanting to appear to be a Luddite, I have felt compelled to explore the question of the doctor/patient relationship. In spite of all the new technology, many patients, and I include the under 30s, yearn for the family doctor who listens, examines, and most of all is empathetic.

We can certainly preserve all these qualities and absorb new technology. We must not throw out 'the baby with the bathwater'. As doctors, we need to remember that we were originally envisaged as a caring profession. If we lose the ability or desire to care for people in their times of distress, then medicine has surely changed.

The Astellas debate, discussed in Chapter 12, raises some of these questions. The answers may become clear in the future.

Shaun R. McCann
May 2015

Acknowledgements

I am extremely grateful to all my colleagues and friends who have given generously of their time to read parts of this book. As a result, the contents should be factually correct, whatever about the writing style. I have listed the names of all those who helped me and, if I have omitted your name and you have helped me, please accept my apologies, as it was a 'sin of omission'. I am grateful to Oxford University Press for accepting my proposal and to Professor Christopher Gardner-Thorpe, the series editor, for his initial approach. Caroline Smith, Senior Assistant Commissioner at Oxford University Press, guided me carefully at every step. I thank Dr Emer Lawlor, Dr Joan O'Riordan, Dr William Murphy, and Dr Diarmuid O'Donghaile, all of whom are from the Irish Blood Transfusion Service. I also thank Dr John Hedley-Whyte, Professor Owen Smith, Professor Paul Browne, Dr Jordi Sierra, Dr Joan Grifols, Professor John Dillon, Dr Clemens Ruthner, Dr Brenda Moore-McCann, Mr James Cogan (artist), Mr Anthony Edwards (photographer), Professor Ian Peake, Professor Lucio Luzzatto, Professor Brian Druker, Professor David Scott, Professor Federico Mingozzi, Dr Darrell Triulzi, Professor Margareta Holström, and Dr Andrea Piccin. Dr Robert Hast provided information on haematology in Sweden, and Professor Mammen Chandy provided information on haematology in India. I would also like to thank Professor Archie Prentice, Professor Robert P. Gale, Ms Mara Neal, the Wallace H. Coulter Foundation, Mr Richard McCafferty, Mr David O'Brien, Professor Sean O'Briain, and Mr Gordon Wright. I am grateful to Professor David McConnell, Professor Yuri Volkov, and Ms Laura Kickham from Trinity College, Dublin, for their help, as well as to Professor Nikolay N. Mamev and Professor Boris V. Afanasyev, who kindly provided me with information on haematology in Russia. I would also like to thank Dr Ronan McDermott, Professor Joseph Harbison, and Dr Brendan Foley from St James' Hospital, Dublin, as well as Professor Peter Voswinckel, who provided information on haematology in Germany.

In addition, I thank Professor Peter Daly for proofreading the final draft. His incisive comments and careful reading were invaluable. I also thank Professors Laurent Degos and Christine Chomienne for their help with the section on APL and Professor Jean Paul Pittion for his helpful advice. Indumadhi Srinivasan and Elizabeth Farrell from Oxford University Press provided excellent guidance and improved the manuscript immeasurably.

Contents

Abbreviations

AAV	Adeno-associated viruses	HDNB	Haemolytic disease of the newborn
ADCM	Automated digital cell morphology	HIT	Heparin-induced thrombocytopenia
AIHA	Autoimmune haemolytic anaemia	HLA	Human leucocyte antigen
APC	Activated Protein C	HS	Hereditary spherocytosis
ASH	American Society of Hematology	HUS	Haemolytic uremic syndrome
		ICSH	International Council for Standardization in Haematology
ATRA	All-trans retinoic acid		
BSH	British Society for Haematology	INSERM	Institute National de la Santé et de la Recherche Médicale
BTK	Bruton's tyrosine kinase		
BTSB	Blood Transfusion Service Board	ISBT	International Society for Blood Transfusion
CAR	Chimaeric antigen receptor	ISH	International Society of Haematology
CD	Cluster of differentiation		
CDB	Center for Developmental Biology	ISHBT	Indian Society of Haematology and Blood Transfusion
CDC	Centers for Disease Control and Prevention	ISTH	International Society on Thrombosis and Haemostasis
CIBMTR	Center for International Blood and Marrow Transplant Research	MHS	Marine Hospital Service
		NIH	National Institutes for Health
		NMDP	National Marrow Donor Program
CNS	Central nervous system		
EBMT	European Society for Blood and Marrow Transplantation	PCI	Percutaneous coronary intervention
EHA	European Haematology Association	PCR-SSO	Sequence-specific oligonucleotide PCR
EPCR	Endothelial Protein C receptor	PCR-SSPs	Sequence-specific primer PCR
EWTD	European Working Time Directive	SNP	Single nucleotide polymorphism
FISH	Fluorescent in situ hybridization	TLR	Toll-like receptor
		TMA	Thrombotic microangiopathy
FITC	Fluorescein isothiocyanate	TTP	Thrombotic thrombocytopenic purpura
G-CSF	Granulocyte colony-stimulating factor	vCJD	Variant Creutzfeldt–Jakob disease
G6PD	Glucose-6-phosphate dehydrogenase	VTE	Venous thromboembolic disease

Chapter 1

Science before science

Introduction

We live in an age of specialization—in fact, super-specialization—which has reached crisis proportions. Although the scientific understanding of many aspects of medicine, and especially haematology, has undoubtedly benefited society, we are now in a position such that few doctors will offer an opinion on anything outside his/her area of sub-specialization. For example, general haematologists will not offer an opinion on coagulation or transfusion medicine problems. Patients suffer, as they may be sent to many different specialists without any doctor taking overall responsibility for their diagnosis and management, even though, as doctors, we must never forget the dictum of Sir William Osler (1849–1919), the famous Canadian physician, who said: 'the good physician treats the disease; the great physician treats the patient who has the disease' (1). What separates us, then, from the classical Greeks, Arab physicians, and the men of the Enlightenment is the fact that they were polymaths, with erudite opinions on many different aspects of natural philosophy and mathematics.

Anybody who writes a book with the word 'history' in the title, in this postmodern age, is bound to evoke controversy. Historians are deeply divided about the definition of the 'Scientific Revolution' and cannot agree on when it began, even if you believe in it as a concept (2). It is now clear that the Dark Ages were not stagnant but it is also true as Cunningham points out (3) that before the 1960s there seemed to be a single interpretation of history: facts were facts. Then, revisionism in history became dominant. Researchers began to unearth new evidence and look at the political and social milieu in which past events took place. 'The facts are really not at all like fish on a fishmongers slab,' according to the English historian E. H. Carr (1892–1982). 'They are like fish swimming about in a vast, sometimes inaccessible, ocean; and what the historian catches will depend, partly on chance, but mainly on what part of the ocean he/she chooses to fish in . . . By and large, the historian will get the kind of facts he/she wants. History means interpretation' (4). Accepting Carr's observation, I shall try to explore the attitudes of the ancients to medicine, but more particularly to blood. In this chapter, I shall concentrate on the history of Western medicine but also mention Chinese, Arab, and Indian medicine, as well as discuss popular legends and myths about blood.

Blood: What is it?

Although haematology is a relatively new specialty in medicine, blood has been of interest since time immemorial. One reason is the relative ease with which one can obtain a sample of blood. When teaching undergraduates, I begin by showing a picture of a tube of anticoagulated blood (Figure 1.1).

The question I ask is: 'What is this?' The answer I usually get is: 'This is a full-blood-count tube of blood.' Incorrect: 'This is a biopsy of a human mesenchymal organ called blood. We can biopsy it daily or more frequently by simply removing a small quantity from a peripheral vein. This ability has undoubtedly led to an understanding of disease mechanisms which have been applied to many other organs.' Molecular medicine, genetics, mechanisms of malignancy, and the understanding of how biochemistry and physiology relate to humans in sickness and health have all been facilitated by the ability to take blood samples easily and frequently.

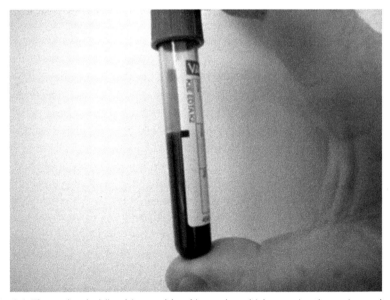

Fig. 1.1 The author holding his own blood in a tube which contains the anticoagulant EDTA.

Bloodletting

Blood, however, was not always taken for investigative reasons. The removal of small quantities of blood from sick individuals as a form of therapy has been known since antiquity. Herodotus (484–425 BC), who was the first Western historian (see cover image), mentions bloodletting (5), as do the Christian Bible (5), and the Talmud (6). Although the ancient Greeks recommended removal of blood (7), the practice was carried out earlier by the Egyptians and probably before that in Mesopotamia. Records (hieroglyphics) from Egypt indicate that cupping, the placing of cups on the skin to apply suction, was undertaken as early as 3500 BC (8). It was also practised in Chinese, Middle Eastern, and Indian cultures. In India, from 1200 to 600 BC, 'raktamokshana', or bloodletting, was practised and is probably still practised in some places today (8).

The idea shared by all these cultures was that removal of blood would restore the internal balance of the bodily humours. Ancient Greek philosophers/physicians believed that humans possessed four humours, termed blood, yellow bile, black bile, and phlegm and whose properties were heat, cold, dryness, and moistness, respectively. These humours were also linked to the four elements air, fire, earth, and water (7). Imbalance of the humours, it was thought, led to disease; this theory was based partly on the idea that menstrual bleeding was a release of 'bad humours'.

Hippocrates (460–377 BC) probably got the idea, at least in part, about the balance of humours and the therapeutic intervention of removing blood to restore that balance, from the Egyptians. The practice of bloodletting was not confined to the Middle East; the earliest record of bloodletting in China comes from Ge Hong in AD 280 (8). Hijama, or cupping, was also practised in Arabia, probably before Muhammad ﷺ (570–630) (8). Bloodletting was also used therapeutically in North America, carried out by the 'medicine man', who was paid a fee for the service and used the small end of a perforated cow's horn to release blood from an infected area.

Extraordinarily, in spite of the experimentation of the Enlightenment and the consequent upsurge in the knowledge of physiology, the practice of bloodletting continued until the end of the nineteenth century. Thomas Jefferson noted in one of his letters that 'in his theory of bleeding and mercury I was ever opposed to my friend Rush [Benjamin Rush], whom I greatly loved. He did much harm, in the sincerest persuasion that he was preserving life and happiness to all around him' (9). Indeed, injudicious bloodletting may have contributed to the death of the first president of the United States, George Washington.

The power of blood

In order to find out what people thought about illness and therapeutics, many Western historians have turned to Herodotus. It is thought that Herodotus was a Greek born in Halicarnassus in present-day Turkey and that he died in Thurii in southern Italy. Later called by Cicero 'the father of history', Herodotus set himself the task of recording the history of the world, something that nobody before him had done, in his famous book called *The Histories*, written almost 500 years before the birth of Christ (10). However, most of *The Histories* was based on stories told to Herodotus during his widespread travels in Egypt, Africa, and throughout Greece. As commented by the Polish journalist Ryszard Kapuściński in his book *Travels with Herodotus*, Herodotus found that each person 'remembers something different—different and differently' and that 'the past does not exist. There are only infinite renderings of it' (11). Therefore, perhaps Herodotus was a revisionist long before that term had been invented.

Nonetheless, Herodotus recounted that the Scythians, who inhabited what we now call Iran from the seventh century BC until the fourth century AD, drank the blood of their slain enemies, using the skulls as drinking vessels (10). I presume this practice would have been based on the belief that the bravery of the slain warrior would be transferred to the victor. Such a belief is not unreasonable, as soldiers died of bleeding from their wounds in battle; so perhaps it was understandable to think that blood contained the quality that gave man 'life'.

Thus, blood was also considered to be a rejuvenating fluid. A famous example of blood being linked to rejuvenation is the Greek myth about the rejuvenation of Jason's father by Medea. There are many versions of the myth about Medea and Jason, but their common theme is that Medea was a sorceress who fell in love with the adventurer Jason. When Jason asked her to reduce his father's age, she slit his father's throat, releasing the old blood; she then infused the blood (some versions say she used ram's blood) with certain herbs and put it back into his body, thus rejuvenating him.

The Scythians were not the only people to drink blood. Although the concept seems strange to us now, the ancient Romans believed that epilepsy could be cured by drinking the blood of a slain gladiator. Pliny the Elder, who lived in the first century AD, tells us: 'Epileptic patients are in the habit of drinking the blood even of gladiators . . . And yet these persons, forsooth, consider it a most effectual cure for their disease, to quaff the warm, breathing, blood from man himself, and, as they apply their mouth to the wound, to draw forth his very life' (12) (see Figure 1.2).

The idea that blood contains something perhaps immeasurable is indicated by repeated commands that prohibit the eating and drinking of blood in the

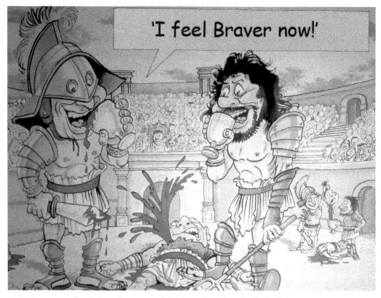

Fig. 1.2 Cartoon depicting Romans drinking the blood of gladiators.

Reproduced by kind permission from James Cogan. Copyright © 2015 James Cogan.

Old Testament, which was probably written in the fifth century BC. In Leviticus 17:11, the phrase 'the life of the flesh is in the blood' suggests that blood contains the soul. In Genesis 9:4 is the admonition 'But you shall not eat flesh with its life, that is, its blood.' Deuteronomy 12:16 states that 'only the blood you must not eat.' And Samuel 1:31–33 reads as follows:

> Now they had driven back the Philistines that day from Michmash to Aijalon. So the people were very faint and the people rushed on the spoil, and took sheep, oxen and calves and slaughtered them on the ground; and the people ate them with the blood. They then told Saul, saying 'Look people are sinning against the Lord by eating with the blood.'[1]

Yet, based on the New Testament account of the Last Supper, Roman Catholics and some other Christian sects believe that wine is converted into the blood of Christ during the Eucharist, to be consumed by the priest and congregation: 'after the same manner also He took the cup, when He supped saying, this cup is the new testament in my blood; this do ye, as oft as ye drink it, in remembrance of me' (13).

Genetics before genetics

Apart from designating the drinking or eating of blood as a sin, the Bible also reveals something about the genetics of bleeding diseases. Since biblical times, observers have commented that some people continued to bleed after relatively minor injury. The Talmud (*c.* AD 200–500) provides insights into the genetics of bleeding disorders that have only been unravelled relatively recently, as there are clear descriptions in the Talmud of bleeding disorders occurring in only males and which were transmitted by apparently 'normal' females. In addition, Rabbi Judah the Patriarch states in the Talmud that, although circumcision was advocated for all male children, the decision to circumcise could be waived if two brothers bled abnormally and died after the event (14). This text is probably the first recorded recognition of the inherited bleeding disorder that occurs only in males and which we now call haemophilia (Figure 1.3).

In 1161, Moses Maimonides (1135–1204), also known as 'Rambam', who was a rabbi, a physician, a philosopher, and a pupil of the philosopher/scientist Averroes, said that, if a woman married a second time, her sons by her second marriage should be exempt from circumcision if any of those from her first had suffered from abnormal bleeding following circumcision (15). He obviously understood, long before genetic studies were undertaken, that an inherited bleeding disorder could be transmitted through the female line. Interestingly, the blood of individuals who exhibited abnormal bleeding was referred to as 'loose' or 'weak' blood.

Another interesting fact is that the book of Genesis states that God commanded Abraham to circumcise all male children on the eighth day after birth. We have known since the 1950s that newborns may be deficient in the fat-soluble vitamin K, which is essential for blood clotting. This vitamin is not present in breast milk but made in the liver and bowel about a week after birth. Thus, newborn babies are now given vitamin K to prevent bleeding in the first few weeks of life. The idea of a relative vitamin deficiency would have been unheard of at the time the book of Genesis was created, but the insight was uncanny: waiting for 8 days after birth before circumcising would minimize the risk of bleeding in children who did not have a congenital coagulopathy.

Pythagoras (570–495 BC), who is best known for his eponymous theorem in geometry, also contributed to haematology. His observations about haematology may have been unintentional but he and many others were familiar with the condition known as 'favism', in which fava beans may cause death if consumed (Figure 1.4). We now know the genetic and biochemical basis of favism: it is caused by a deficiency of the enzyme glucose-6-phosphate dehydrogenase. This

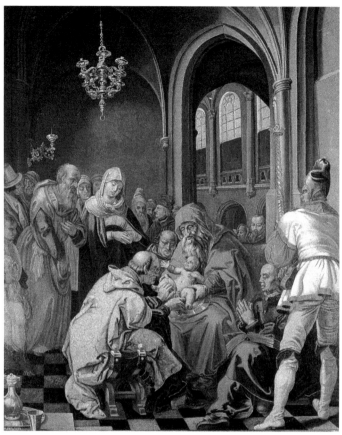

Fig. 1.3 *The Circumcision of Christ*; oil painting after Hendrik Goltzius.

Reproduced from Wellcome Library, London. Image ID: L0005695. Library reference no.: ICV No 17752. Copyright © 2015 Wellcome Library, London, UK.

deficiency is an hereditary trait prevalent in countries in the Mediterranean basin. If an affected individual eats fava beans (or even inhales fava bean pollen), acute intravascular haemolysis (premature red cell death) results, presumably secondary to oxidative stress, and the individual becomes jaundiced and very unwell.

The genetic basis for the enzyme deficiency was not unravelled until the twentieth century; however, G6PD deficiency remains the most common of all enzyme abnormalities in man. The disease is X-linked, and Pythagoras had enough insight to forbid his followers to eat fava beans. The fact that his followers were all male may have been fortuitous. According to John Meletis, writing in the *Archives of Hellenic Medicine*, Pythagoras was killed by his enemies from

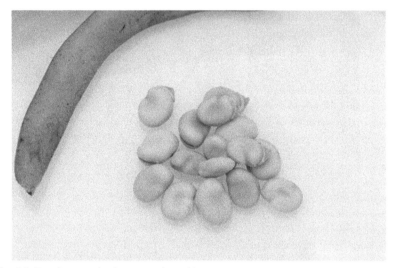

Fig. 1.4 Fava beans, also known as broad beans.

Reproduced by kind permission of Shaun McCann. Copyright © 2015 Shaun McCann.

Crotonia because he refused to cross a field of fava beans (16). Meletis also quotes Iamblichus, a Syrian philosopher/neoplatonist (245–325), as stating that a number of disciples of Pythagoras were slaughtered while fleeing from their enemies because they refused to cross a field of fava beans (16).

Historical views of the circulatory system

One Greek who had a huge influence on Western medicine was Hippocrates (460–370 BC), who was from Cos and is often referred to as 'the father of Western medicine' (7). Hippocrates' theory of the four humours (hot and dry-yellow bile, cold and dry-black bile, cold and wet-phlegm, and hot and wet-blood), as well the idea that imbalance between these humours caused disease and that therefore removing small quantities of blood might restore balance to a sick individual, would influence medicine for hundreds of years.

Nonetheless, Hippocrates and his followers were hampered in their quest for knowledge of human anatomy and physiology by the fact that, in the cities where they lived, human dissection was forbidden; hence, many of their observations were extrapolated from animal studies and human embryos. However, two other Greeks, Erasistratus (304–250 BC) and his colleague Herophilus (335–280 BC), were accomplished anatomists who worked in Alexandria, where human dissection was not forbidden. The fact that the tradition in Alexandria was Ptolemaic, in other words Egyptian, may account for the different attitude to human dissection, as there was a long tradition of anatomical science in Egypt. Some of their dissections were performed in public and it is said that Erasistratus was so enthusiastic that he even dissected living criminals. He probably described what we now call the tricuspid valve and came very close to an accurate description of the systemic and pulmonary circulation. Although most of the writings of Erasistratus have not survived, some were preserved by Galen (c.129–210), another Greek who had a huge influence on Western medicine (7).

Galen, who was from Pergamum, was reputed to have been a forceful and domineering personality and was one of the most prolific writers of all time (7). Based on the observations of Erasistratus, he wrote of the circulatory system that 'the vein arises from the part where the arteries, which are distributed to the whole body, have their origin, and penetrates to the right ventricle; the pulmonary vein arises from the part where veins have their origin, and penetrates to the left ventricle of the heart.' This description is close to what Ibn al-Nafis and Harvey would write hundreds of years later.

However, like Hippocrates and his followers, Galen was unable to conduct detailed studies of human anatomy and so many of his ideas about the circulatory system were extrapolated. For example, he disagreed with some of the basic anatomical descriptions of the heart by Erasistratus, in particular that the heart was a pump; instead, he believed that blood passed from the right to the left side of the heart through small holes. He also disagreed with Erasistratus and Herophilus that veins carried blood and that arteries carried pneuma, soul, or spirit. Many of Galen's ideas were based on Hippocrates' theory of the four humours, and he believed that the liver was the main site of blood production (17); it took 700 years before doubts began to appear about his medical theories.

Haematology in the Islamic Golden Age

Were there any developments in medicine from the time of Galen until the Enlightenment? Yes—in the so-called Islamic Golden Age, which stretched from the eighth to the sixteenth centuries. It is important to understand that, under the Abbasid Caliphate (750–1258), Muslim scholars had access to Greco-Roman, Byzantine, Indian, Egyptian, and Persian civilizations and were aware of many things that Western scholars only came to know in the late Middle Ages. The development of the 'scientific method' in the Arab world, for example, occurred in the eighth century, preceding the Enlightenment by hundreds of years.

Arab scholars, physicians, and philosophers were undoubtedly influenced by Galen and his Greek colleagues, but a number of important insights were also supplied by Arab physicians/philosophers. Influential centres in the Islamic Golden Age were Baghdad, Damascus, and Cairo (7).

Galen's teachings were challenged by many Arab philosopher/physicians during the Islamic Golden Age, when the Arab empire stretched from Spain to Persia, including Avicenna (Ibn Sina; 980–1037), a Persian polymath who wrote mainly in Arabic, and Ibn al-Nafis, an Arab physician (1213–88). Avicenna's work *The Canon of Medicine*, which was based on the teachings of Galen and Hippocrates, was used as a textbook in Western universities, presumably in translation, for over 500 years after his death. Later on, in the thirteenth century, Ibn al-Nafis was a practising physician who studied medicine in Damascus and was attached to the Mansuri Hospital in Cairo. In his commentary on Avicenna's *Canon of Medicine*, Ibn al-Nafis clearly describes the pulmonary circulation, although there is still reference to blood mixing with air to become 'purified' (7) (Figure 1.5).

Ibn al-Nafis, a product of the intellectual environment of the Mamluk dynasty, lived through a time of great political upheaval including the Christian

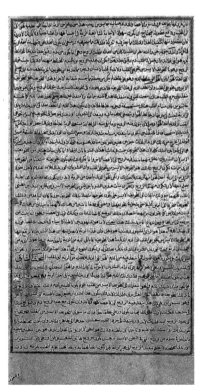

Fig. 1.5 Photo of a page from Ibn al-Nafis's *Commentary on Anatomy in Avicenna's Canon*, which contains the first description of the pulmonary circulation.

Reproduced from Wellcome Library, London. Image ID: L0030233. Library reference no.: MS OR 51. Copyright © 2015 Wellcome Library, London, UK.

Crusades, the victories of Saladin, and the Mongol threat. Unfortunately, no extant contemporary source mentions him. This omission may be due to professional jealousy, political patronage, religious rivalry, or a combination of all three. In addition, Ibn al-Nafis wrote in Arabic and well before the arrival of the printing press in the fifteenth century, so his writings would have been difficult to reproduce in the West. All of these reasons may have contributed to the almost total exclusion of his work on pulmonary circulation from the canon (18).

In addition, Ibn al-Nafis was concerned with a physiology that relied heavily on Aristotle's hylomorphism, which stated that 'being' was a combination of matter and form (19). Ibn al-Nafis emphasized the purity and fineness of the spirit and suggested that as blood was mixed with air in the lungs it became very fine and passed to the left side of the heart from where it was converted into the 'spirit' and then cooled and thickened in the brain. Nonetheless, it is clear that he refuted the Galenic theory that blood passes from the right side to the left side of the heart through tiny septae.

Haematology in the fifteenth century and during the Enlightenment

While physicians in the Arab world kept the ideas of Galen alive, although modified and embellished, it wasn't until 1553 that a clear description of pulmonary circulation was published in the West, in *Christianismi Restitutio*, written by Michael Servetus (1511–53), a polymath Spanish physician and Humanist. However, as his book was a religious treatise, it was not widely read in medical/scientific circles. It did not help that most copies were burnt, as was Servetus, as a heretic. Western understanding of the human body and disease did not really alter until the writings of people like Vesalius (1514–64), who was a Belgian physician and anatomist. His detailed anatomical studies and illustrations in *De Humani Corporis Fabrica* made this information widely available. However, as there were 273 illustrations in that book, it is very unlikely that they were all drawn by one person, and some of them may have been made by Jan Stephen van Calcar (a pupil of Titian) and his followers; nonetheless, Vesalius' reputation as an anatomist persists (20). Other European scholars who challenged Galen's work include Realdus Columbus (1516–59), who was an Italian surgeon and anatomist, Juan Valverde de Amusco (1525–87), who was a Spanish doctor and anatomist, and William Harvey (1578–1657), an English physician.

It should also be remembered that people like Boyle, Harvey, Newton, and other philosopher/scientists of the Enlightenment believed in magic while at the same time pursuing scientific experimentation. In addition, these men believed in a divine God, and their efforts to understand nature by their experiments and observations were fundamentally investigations into the way God created the natural world (2, 21). Nonetheless, modern medicine and haematology began, in earnest, during the Enlightenment. The publications by Harvey, the experiments in England and France with blood transfusion, and the discovery and use of the microscope by doctors were all necessary for progress in the understanding of blood diseases and subsequently for their treatment.

Although many experiments were carried out in England and France to try to understand the circulation of the blood, an accurate anatomical description of the pulmonary circulation had been around for many years, as the illustrations of Ibn al-Nafis show very clearly (Figure 1.5). In spite of this, in almost every text to this day, Harvey gets the credit for this discovery. Like most discoveries, however, many ideas of a similar nature often preceded that of the person credited by historians. It should be remembered that Harvey had studied Galen's medicine while at Cambridge University in the late sixteenth century. We do not know if Harvey was familiar with the writings of either Ibn al-Nafis or Avicenna. His failure to refer to either may be because of difficulty in gaining access to medical treatises, an inability to read Arabic, or perhaps a degree of prejudice.

The idea of using blood as a therapeutic intervention, however, could not have been developed without an understanding of the circulatory system. The evolution of transfusion medicine was far from a smooth affair, as we will see, and it took a long time, even after the establishment of the systemic and pulmonary circulations, before blood transfusion became widely accepted.

Haematology and traditional Chinese medicine

Did traditional Chinese medicine make a significant contribution to haematology? In recent years, the extremely important discoveries that acute promyelocytic leukaemia could be treated and probably cured with the carboxylic acid form of vitamin A (all-trans retinoic acid) and that arsenic trioxide (As_2O_3) could be used to treat relapse were made in China (22, 23). Tantalizingly, in the Yellow Emperor's *Classic on Internal Medicine*, which was probably written in the second century BC, there is a description of what sounds very like the circulation: 'The blood current flows continuously in a circle and never stops.' Once again, we can see that other people had the idea of blood circulating long before Harvey did. Otherwise, there is not much evidence that blood diseases were considered important in ancient Chinese medicine. However, the Chinese seem to have taken examination of the pulse to extremes: the medical treatise *Muo-Ching* (composed in 152–219) comprised ten volumes about the intricacies of the pulse (8) (Figure 1.6).

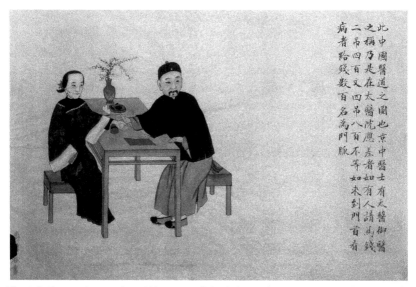

Fig. 1.6 Photo of an ancient Chinese scroll depicting a doctor examining the pulse of his patient.

Reproduced from Wellcome Library, London. Image ID: L0004700. Library reference no.: Slide number 7383. Copyright © 2015 Wellcome Library, London, UK.

Haematology in traditional Indian medicine (Ayurvedic medicine)

Apart from therapeutic bloodletting, termed 'raktamokshana', there is little mention of blood or blood diseases in ancient Indian medicine, although malaria was a problem. Interestingly, in a fashion similar to that of the classical Greeks, Ayurvedic practitioners enumerate five bodily substances: earth, water, fire, air, and aether. They also recognize seven basic tissues: plasma, blood, muscles, bone, marrow, fat, and semen (8).

The vampire legend and *Dracula*

There is probably no legend that has fired the human imagination more than that of the vampire. The connection between blood, the 'undead', and sex has gripped people's fantasies, perhaps as no other story ever did. A famous, fascinating, and early legend connected to drinking blood is that of Countess Elizabeth Báthory de Ecsed (1560–1614) in Slovakia. She was reputed to have drunk and bathed in the blood of virgins to retain her youth (24). Her story may have influenced the writings of Bram Stoker 300 years later and perhaps she served as a model for the wicked queen in the Grimm Brothers' fairy tale 'Snow White'. She was imprisoned and died in Csejte (Čachice) castle, in Slovakia.

In the early eighteenth century, a combination of war and infectious diseases stimulated the modern interest in the vampire legends of the Balkan areas that had recently been recaptured by the Austrian military. At that time, there were many outbreaks of plague and typhus. Outbreaks of these infectious diseases may have stimulated hysteria about vampires because of the abnormal bleeding associated with them. Christian Reiter, a forensic pathologist from the University of Vienna, has recently argued that a number of deaths in the Serbian village of Medvegia in 1731–2, attributed to vampirism, were actually caused by anthrax rather than vampirism. However, it may be that these infections were complicated by disseminated intravascular coagulation and thus led to bleeding into the skin, mouth, nose, brain, or other internal organs. Critically, after death, blood may have continued to escape from the mouth and nose and have been misinterpreted as fresh bleeding (25).

The paradigm for the modern vampire, a handsome aristocrat seducing beautiful young girls, evolved from a publication entitled *The Vampyre: A Tale*, written by John Polidori, a medical doctor, in 1819. However it was the novel *Carmilla*, written in 1872 by Sheridan le Fanu, and later Bram Stoker's *Dracula*, written in 1897, which promulgated the popularity of the vampire myth in Europe (26, 27). Le Fanu undoubtedly influenced Bram Stoker. Stoker may also have been inspired by the Victorian writer Emily Gerard, who in 1885 wrote an essay on Transylvanian superstitions, noting that the legend of the Nosferatu or vampire was widely believed in Transylvania.

It is obvious that Stoker had some knowledge of haematology. In his novel, the character Lucy, who becomes anaemic because of repeated blood sucking by Dracula, requires a blood transfusion. Professor Van Helsing is summoned and decides, with the local doctor John Seward, that 'there is no time to be lost. She will die for sheer want of blood to keep the heart's action as it should be. There must be transfusion of blood at once.' Thus, Stoker understood the possibility of heart failure from severe anaemia; he also understood the technique of blood transfusion, as Van Helsing says of Arthur, Lucy's fiancé: 'He is so young and strong and of blood so pure that we need not defibrinate it.' Stoker, however, clearly knew nothing about blood groups and could not have been aware of the possibility of severe and fatal transfusion reactions, since on a number of occasions he uses different donors for Lucy. In spite of his medical knowledge and scientific training, Van Helsing also states that 'a brave man's blood is the best thing on this earth when a woman is in trouble.' Like the ancients, Stoker believed that the 'character' of the donor was in some way present in blood and that a brave man's blood was different to that of a coward.

Some modern film-makers and novelists have inverted the vampire myth by making vampires the dominant species, incorporating the possibility of a shortage of human blood, and some contemporary performance artists have made their names by self-mutilation and drawing blood. The vampire stories were chilling, especially in the nineteenth century, and the so-called magic properties of blood continue to fascinate. Yet blood, first and foremost, is a biological fluid, which carries oxygen, carbon dioxide, a number of clotting proteins, red and white cells, and platelets. Although, as in *Dracula*, a red cell transfusion can be life-saving, vampirism remains, as it always was, a myth.

References

1 **Bliss M**. William Osler: A Life in Medicine. First edition. Oxford University Press, New York, NY, 1999.

2 **Henry J**. The Scientific Revolution and the Origin of Modern Science. Second edition. Studies in European History. Palgrave, London, 2002.

3 **Cunningham A, Williams P**. De-centring the 'big picture': *The Origin of Modern Science* and the modern origins of science. British Journal of the History of Science **26**(4): 407–32. 1993.

4 **Carr EH**. What Is History? Cambridge University Press, Cambridge, 1961.

5 **Riches J**. The Bible: A Very Short Introduction. Oxford University Press, Oxford, 2000.

6 **Rosner F**. Bloodletting in Talmudic times: Bulletin of the New York Academy of Medicine **62**(9): 935–46. 1986.

7 **Bynum W**. The History of Medicine: A Very Short Introduction. Oxford University Press, Oxford, 2008.

8 **Lyons AS, Petrucelli RJ**. Medicine: An Illustrated History. Harry N. Abrams, New York, NY, 1987.

9 **Binger C**. Revolutionary Doctor Benjamin Rush, 1746–1813. W. W Norton, New York, NY, 1966.

10 **Herodotus**. The Histories. Revised edition. Penguin Classics. Penguin Books, New York, NY, 1972.

11 **Kapuściński R**. Travels with Herodotus. Penguin Books, New York, NY, 2008.

12 **Knapp R**. Invisible Romans. Profile Books Ltd, London, 2011.

13 The New King James Version. Thomas Nelson, Nashville, TN, 1982.

14 **Jacobs J, Fishberg M**. 'Morbidity', in JewishEncyclopedia: The Unedited Full-text of the Jewish Encyclopedia, 1906. http://jewishencyclopedia.com/articles/10982-morbidity, 2011.

15 **Rosner F**. The Medical Legacy of Moses Maimonides. KTAV Publishing House, Jersey City, NJ, 1998.

16 **Meletis J**. Favism: A brief history from the "abstain from beans" of Pythagoras to the present. Archives of Hellenic Medicine **29**(2): 258–63. 2012.

17 **Galen**. On the Usefulness of the Parts of the Body [De Usu Partium]. Translated from the Greek with an Introduction and Commentary by Margaret Tallmadge May. Cornell University Press, Ithaca, NY, 1968.

18 **West JB**. Ibn al-Nafis, the pulmonary circulation, and the Islamic Golden Age. Journal of Applied Physiology **105**(6): 1877–80. 2008.

19 **Fancy H**. Science and Religion in Mamluk Egypt: Ibn al-Nafis, Pulmonary Transit and Bodily Resurrection. Routledge, Milton Park, 2013.

20 **Williamson G**. 'Jan Stephanus van Kalcker', in The Catholic Encyclopedia (1913), Vol 8. https://en.wikisource.org/wiki/Catholic_Encyclopedia_%281913%29/Jan_Stephanus_van_Kalcker, 2013.

21 **Butterfield H**. The Origins of Modern Science. Revised edition. The Free Press, New York, NY, 1997.

22 **Huang ME, Ye YC, Chen SR, Chai JR, Lu JX, Zhoa L, et al**. Use of all-trans retinoic acid in the treatment of acute promyelocytic leukemia. Blood **72**(2): 567–72. 1988.

23 **Shen ZX, Chen GQ, Ni JH, Li XS, Xiong SM, Qiu QY, et al**. Use of arsenic trioxide (As_2O_3) in the treatment of acute promyelocytic leukemia (APL): II. Clinical efficacy and pharmacokinetics in relapsed patients. Blood **89**(9): 3354–60. 1997.

24 **Craft KL**. The Infamous Lady: The True Story of Countess Erzsebét Báthory. First edition. CreateSpace Independent Publishing Platform, North Charleston, SC, 2009.

25 **Reiter C**. Der Vampyr-Aberglaube und die Militärärzte. http://www.kakanien.ac.at/beitr/Vamp/CReiter1, 2007.

26 **Le Fanu S**. Carmilla. DODO Press, Gloucester, 2009.

27 **Stoker B**. Dracula. Oxford University Press, Oxford, 2011.

Chapter 2

The Enlightenment and the unravelling of the circulation

Blood beliefs

Many qualities other than being a tissue which is necessary for life have been attributed to blood. Kinship (blood brothers), class (blue blood, royal blood), and even emotional states (boiling blood) have been attributed to this fluid. In antiquity, blood sacrifice was perceived as the ultimate offering to the gods. The Bible recounts that Abel used blood sacrifice and found favour with God (1). The pre-Columbian Aztecs cut out the hearts of living victims to ensure the perpetuation of the world (2). Probably the most dramatic example at the present time is the belief, shared by Roman Catholics, Copts, and Orthodox Christians, that wine is transubstantiated into the blood of Christ by the priest during celebration of the Eucharist.

The Enlightenment and the first blood transfusion experiments

There is disagreement among historians regarding the beginning of the Enlightenment; it may have been ushered in with René Descartes (1596–1650) in 1637 or with Isaac Newton (1642–1726/7) in 1688. Against the backdrop of logic, reason, empiricism, and direct experimentation and observation, the philosopher/scientist William Harvey's (1578–1657) written description of the circulation of the blood opened the floodgates of scientific research and discovery (3). Harvey, the eldest of nine siblings, graduated with a BA from Gonville and Ciaus College in Cambridge and in 1602 received his medical diploma in Padua. He returned to England and graduated as a doctor from Cambridge. He was elected a Fellow of the Royal Society in 1607. In 1615 he began to make his views about the pulmonary circulation known in a series of lectures at the College of Physicians (Figure 2.1). Harvey (Figure 2.2) suggested that the heart acted as a pump that propelled blood around the body and that it returned to the heart via a system of one-way valves (Figure 2.3); his work had been made possible by the prior work of Vesalius (1514–64), Colombo (1515–99) and Ibn al-Nafis (1213–88). Erastratus (304–250 BC), in Alexandria, had also described

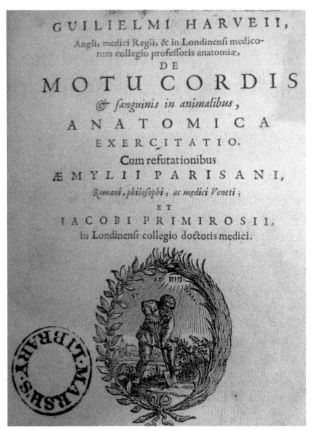

Fig. 2.1 Frontispiece of the 1649 edition of *De Motu Cordis*.

the heart as a pump, and the ancient Chinese understood that blood circulated around the body. However, it was not until the seventeenth century that the idea that blood could be transfused from one animal to another seems to have occurred to physicians.

Harvey's work encouraged further questioning, research, and discovery, although many colleagues and philosophers tried to discredit him. However famous philosophers, many of whom were members of the Royal Society, such as Christopher Wren (1632–1723) and Robert Boyle (1627–91), were intrigued by Harvey's description and its implications. The English philosopher Francis Bacon (1561–1626), for example, developed a laboratory to conduct scientific experiments; but it was the Oxford experiments of Richard Lower (1631–91)

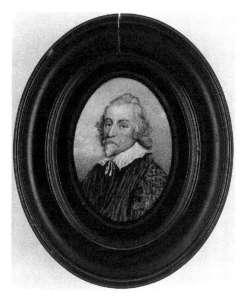

Fig. 2.2 A portrait of William Harvey.

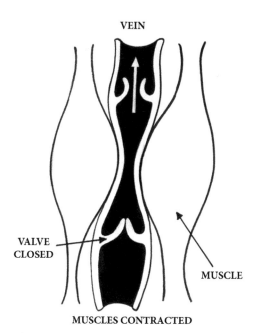

Fig. 2.3 One-way valves showing blood travelling in one direction, that is, towards the heart.

which applied Harvey's ideas and stimulated the progress of blood transfusion. Lower was a surgeon/anatomist and described in detail how to transfuse blood between dogs by using neck veins connected by silver tubes. These experiments failed, as the blood clotted. In 1666, however, he had some success. He bled a dog until it was moribund and then, having exposed a large artery in the neck of another dog, he placed a reed between the artery and vein and blood flowed into the moribund dog. He described how tying the jugular vein was safe and that the dog could survive with one jugular vein. The dog leaped from the table, shook himself, and then ran away as if nothing had happened (4).

Robert Boyle, also a Fellow of the Royal Society, proposed a number of questions for Lower, including whether a dog's disposition could be altered by blood transfusions; in other words, could a dog lose its acquired habit of fetching and carrying or 'dive after ducks' (5)? What intrigues us now are the philosophical questions raised by these experiments, namely, the possibility of transferring acquired characteristics from one animal or human to another. These questions reflected the view that blood contained spirits that could possibly be transferred from one individual to another, a belief dating back to the Greeks or even earlier.

Did these serious thinkers really believe that blood contained spirits and that its transfusion could alter behaviour of the recipient? Apparently they did; but they also believed that blood could be transfused from animals into man. In 1667, at a meeting of the Royal Society, Lower transfused blood from a sheep into the arm vein of Arthur Coga in the belief that the mental health of the latter could be improved by this process. The transfusion lasted for a few minutes, and no untoward effects were recorded. Although described as a volunteer, Coga was paid 20 shillings, a significant amount of money in those days, to undergo the experiment (6). Soon, scientific competition and jealousy became evident. The Royal Society in England, founded shortly before the French Academy of Science in 1660, probably contributed to the competition, according to Holly Tucker's book *Blood Work*. She goes into detail about the rivalry between England and France, citing the work of Jean-Baptiste Denys (1643–1704), a Montpellier graduate who worked at the court of King Louis XIV of France (1638–1715). Perhaps having read of Lower's experiments (7), Denys, in association with a surgeon, Paul Emmerez, performed a number of dog-to-dog transfusions. He also carried out a blood transfusion from a lamb to a young boy in 1667, reportedly without causing ill effects (Figure 2.4). Denys conducted a number of animal-to-human transfusions and submitted a report to the Royal Society in July 1667. Publication was delayed, however, until September because the editor of the journal was imprisoned in the Tower of London!

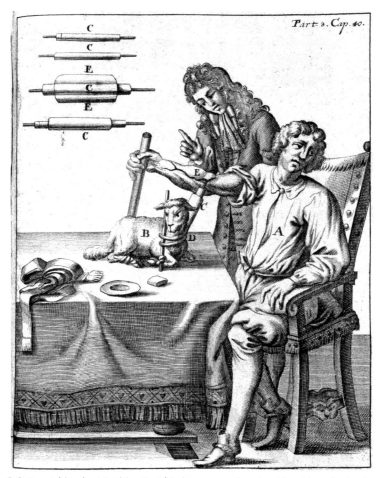

Fig. 2.4 An etching by Matthias Gottfried Purmann showing blood transfusion from a lamb into a man (1705).

Denys went on to carry out probably the most notorious animal-to-human transfusion, one which was to undermine the reputation of blood transfusion. He recommended blood transfusion from a calf as treatment for a man who appeared to be mentally disturbed. The description of what happened after the transfusion was obviously a haemolytic transfusion reaction: back pain, intravascular haemolysis, and haemoglobinuria (7). The patient died following a further attempt at transfusion. It later transpired that the patient's wife had poisoned him with arsenic; however, by that point the reputation of blood transfusion in

France had been severely damaged. Eleven years later, the French Parliament deemed transfusion a criminal act (7). The Royal Society soon followed suit and began to distance itself from blood transfusion, and the following year Pope Innocent XI (1629–91) banned the practice (7).

It is curious that these seventeenth-century physicians advocated blood transfusion not as a way to counteract blood loss but rather as a way to correct characteristics in the recipient, such as mental illness; some even suggested that marital disharmony might be cured by transfusions between spouses (4). Thus, although the idea that blood could cure maladies was discussed by philosophers/physicians, blood transfusion as a means of replacing blood loss or following war injuries had to wait a number of centuries before being recognized as an acceptable treatment.

Post-partum haemorrhage: The penny drops!

Almost 150 years after the banning of blood transfusion, James Blundell (1790–1877), a Scottish obstetrician sometimes referred to as the 'father of modern blood transfusion', performed the first human-to-human blood transfusion in 1818. He was particularly concerned with post-partum haemorrhage and so revived blood transfusion as a possible solution. He published an account of the first successful blood transfusion to a woman with post-partum haemorrhage in *The Lancet* in 1829 (8). He also made the prescient observation that blood transfusion might be used to save the lives of wounded soldiers. Robert McDonnell (1828–89) reported a human-to-human blood transfusion in 1870 in *The Dublin Quarterly Journal of Medical Science* (9). He transfused his own blood, after filtering it, into a 14-year-old girl suffering major trauma, using what we would consider today to be a rather quaint apparatus (Figure 2.5). There were no ill effects of the transfusion but, unfortunately, the patient died

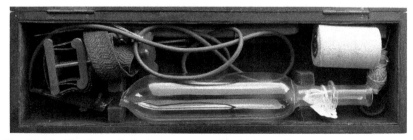

Fig. 2.5 The blood transfusion apparatus used by McDonnell.

the following day. McDonnell advocated the use of blood transfusion for blood loss, chlorosis, and cholera, among other ailments.

Human blood for humans

In the latter part of the nineteenth century, two different German doctors, Emil Ponfick (1844–1913 AD) and Leonard Landois (1837–1902), argued that blood should not be transfused from one species to another. This hypothesis was crucial to the development of safe blood transfusion, finally put an end to animal-to-human transfusions, and cleared the way for less extreme ideas about blood transfusion. Then, reflecting an important cultural change of attitude, during the Franco-Prussian war (1870–1) blood transfusion was advocated as a potential solution to the blood loss suffered by wounded soldiers. Unfortunately for the latter, the suggestion did not become a practical reality. Finally, the discoveries of Louis Pasteur (1822–95) and Joseph Lister (1827–1912) contributed to the story of blood transfusion when they showed that bacteria and fungi could be transmitted as infectious agents from one individual to another and that sterilization of transfusion instruments was vital in preventing such spread.

Blood groups: Yes, they are important

In order to make blood transfusion safe, the biology of the blood groups needed to be understood. Karl Landsteiner (1868–1943) discovered the major blood groups in 1901 and recognized the possibility of a fatal reaction if different blood types were mixed in a patient. Six years later, Ludvig Hekoten (1863–1951) in Chicago recommended testing the blood groups of recipient and prospective donor and crossmatching them before transfusion. Another 6 years were to pass before Reuben Ottenberg (1882–1959), in New York, conclusively proved the necessity for crossmatching before transfusion by showing that antibodies in patients' blood could be harmful to donors' red cells. Since these early days, many further minor blood groups have been discovered, and this knowledge has contributed immensely to the fields of forensic science and anthropology. A lot of confusion existed, initially, because of different nomenclatures for the major blood groups; it was not until 1927 that the A/B/O nomenclature became widely accepted.

In 1914 Albert Hustin (1882–1967), in Brussels, and Luis Agote (1868–1954), in Buenos Aires, discovered that blood clotting could be stopped by the addition of the calcium chelator sodium citrate. In 1916 Peyton Rous and J. R. Turner, together in the Rockefeller Institute in New York produced a solution of glucose and citrate which stopped blood from clotting and allowed the red cells to stay alive for a few weeks. This finding was a very important development, as it opened the door for the storage of blood and the creation of blood banks (10, 11).

Oh, What a Lovely War!

Oh, What a Lovely War! is an anti-war musical film directed by Richard Attenborough in 1969, based on a musical play of the same name, which satirizes the conduct of World War I.

Many changes in medical practice have been instigated by war; nonetheless, in spite of the carnage of World War I, there doesn't seem to have been a large usage of blood transfusion during that war. However, two people, Captain Oswald Hope Robertson, from Harvard Medical School, and Major Lawrence Bruce Robertson, a Toronto surgeon, made significant contributions. As Stansbury and Hess point out in their fascinating article (12), the two Robertsons are often confused and their careers conflated. The Canadians and Americans were ahead of the British in terms of blood transfusion but one of the American pioneers of transfusion, George W. Crile, is now almost forgotten. Crile was convinced as early as 1898 that the fluid of choice for the treatment of haemorrhagic shock was blood (13). The attitude of the medical profession in Britain to blood transfusion in the early twentieth century is obvious from an editorial in the *British Medical Journal* in response to an article by Crile: 'Excellent results were certainly obtained in some cases of shock, but in the treatment of this condition, and indeed, of all others in which intravascular transfusion of some kind is clearly indicated, surgeons, we imagine, will find no good reason given here for abandoning the safe and simple method of saline injections' (14). L. B. Robertson learned the syringe technique of direct blood transfusion from Edward Lindeman at Bellevue Hospital in New York; after he arrived in France in September 1915, he reported four blood transfusions, including one death from haemolysis. His was the first article on wartime blood transfusion in the twentieth century (15). Although O. H. Robertson did not arrive in France until May 1917, his diaries are particularly poignant: 'We were simply deluged . . . hemorrhage, hemorrhage—blood everywhere—clothes soaked in blood, pools of blood in the stretchers, streams of blood dropping from the stretchers to the floor . . . I could transfuse an occasional one but the majority had to take their chances without much treatment and go thru operation as best they could provided there was any possibility at all of their standing operation' (16). The importance of O. H. Robertson's work was that blood could be transfused to wounded soldiers at the battlefront long before they were transported to safety. O. H. Robertson developed the transfusion bottle, demonstrated the use and safety of stored universal donor or crossmatched blood, and enjoyed a long academic career during which he received the Landsteiner Award of the American Association of Blood Banks in 1958 (16). In 1922 Geoffrey Keynes wrote: 'The first transfusion of citrated blood was performed by L. Agote of Buenos Aires on November 1914, but despite this, transfusion of blood was considered to be too difficult and unsuited for the stress of war conditions until 1917' (17).

The next step took some time to come but was significant in that it attempted to establish better systems on a larger scale than before. Alexander Bogdanov (1873–1928), a founder of Bolshevism, was also a physician, economist, philosopher, and poet. In 1926 he persuaded Joseph Stalin to provide funding for the first institute of blood transfusion in the world and carried out many transfusion experiments in the institute. Although he recognized the great potential of blood replacement in war to save lives, he also believed, like many before him, that blood contained a special substance and that the benefits of blood transfusion were much more complex than volume replacement and restoration of oxygen-carrying capacity. Bogdanov thought that blood transfusion could inhibit the ageing process, a belief that goes back to ancient times. He died prematurely, probably from a blood transfusion reaction, but he had managed to establish clearly the basis for a centralized blood transfusion service in the Soviet Union (18). Meanwhile, two other Russians, Vladimir Shamov and the surgeon Sergei Yudin, pioneered the use of blood donation from dead people (cadaveric blood). Although the practice never gained popularity in the former Soviet Union or anywhere else, they made major contributions to the technology of the preservation of donated blood.

Apart from these developments, not much happened in terms of breakthroughs in transfusion science between the end of the Great War and the 1930s. Percy Lane Oliver, a London librarian with an altruistic personality, did manage, however, to set up the first volunteer panel of blood donors in 1921. His efforts were opposed by many doctors because of lingering doubts about the benefits and safety of blood transfusion. Oliver's ideas, however, eventually led to the formation of the British Red Cross Blood Transfusion Service and ultimately to the national Blood Transfusion Service.

The Spanish Civil War: The birth of modern blood transfusion?

The men who made a significant difference to blood transfusion in the modern era were a Canadian, Henry Norman Bethune (1890–1939), and a Spaniard, Frederick Durán-Jordà (1905–57). Bethune was a member of the communist party in Montreal. In the monograph published by the American Society of

Hematology in 2009, *50 Years in Hematology*, Bethune is not mentioned; this omission shows perhaps that one's political outlook can sometimes decide whether or not you are included in the historical record.

Bethune contracted pulmonary tuberculosis and, like many others, thought he was going to die. According to Ted Allan and Sydney Gordon in their book *The Scalpel and the Sword*, he read about the technique of surgical collapse of the lung and insisted on having the procedure carried out (19). He made a full recovery. He was a spendthrift and, according to a relative, Don Bethune (Norman was a cousin of Don's grandfather), 'Norman was very eccentric and he drove my grandmother nuts when he would visit them at their (farm) called "Lindores", named after the small town the Bethune's came from in Fife near Loch Lindores in Scotland. Every time he needed money, for a cause, he would ask my grandparents and they were happy to give it to him' (20). When Norman believed he was dying from tuberculosis, he told his wife she should divorce him and start a new life. She did. Bethune believed in the association between social deprivation and illness, and particularly between poverty and tuberculosis, ideas not widely held by the medical profession. He was equally influenced at a medical conference in Leningrad in the summer of 1935 by the idea that treatment was a 'right of the individual, and not a charity'.

In 1936 he was invited by the Committee to Aid Spanish Democracy (CASD), which was dedicated to raising money to support the Republican cause, to lead a surgical team to Spain to care for the wounded. By all accounts, Bethune was a rather difficult man who did not like taking orders and hated dealing with administrators, but he pursued the idea of a centralized blood bank in Madrid, from where blood could be dispatched to the war front, and saw it as a Canadian contribution to the Republican cause (Figure 2.6).

In 1937 Bethune wrote a poem, 'Red Moon' (21), which contained the lines:

Above the shattered Spanish troops
Last night rose low and wild and red
Reflecting back from her illuminated shield
The blood bespattered faces of the dead . . . [1]

He got funding from CASD for a station wagon, an incubator, a fridge, and an autoclave and thereby established the new transfusion service. He was soon made the director of the blood transfusion service in the Medical School in Madrid, with a team including two Spanish physicians and a Canadian driver, as well as technicians, nurses, and administrative staff. Blood donors were recruited via radio and newspapers, with great success. Donors were given extra

---

[1] Reproduced from Canadian Forum 17.198 (July 1937): 118.

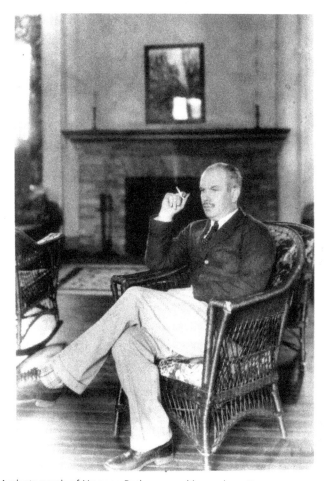

Fig. 2.6 A photograph of Norman Bethune smoking a cigarette.

Reproduced with kind permission from the Royal College of Physicians of Edinburgh. Copyright © 2015 Royal College of Physicians of Edinburgh.

food ration cards in return for donating as often as three times weekly. A mobile transfusion service across a 1000 km front was developed and, crucially, Bethune recognized the importance of transfusing casualties early, before they were transported behind the lines to a hospital. Sadly, as the service developed, Bethune himself became more irascible. It appears that he drank heavily and committed a number of sexual indiscretions. Eventually, he decided that the Republicans' desire to control the transfusion service and his free spirit were incompatible. So he returned to Canada, leaving a whiff of political scandal and an accusation of spying lingering in the air. In spite of this, he conducted a very successful lecture tour in Canada and raised money for the transfusion service in Spain. Bethune subsequently emigrated to China to work for Mao Zedong, eventually dying of blood poisoning from a cut sustained during surgery. He is buried in the Revolutionary Martyrs' Cemetery, Shijiazhuang, in Hebei Province and is regarded as a hero in China.

While it is true that, by 1937, the first blood bank in the United States had already been established (by the Hungarian physician Bernard Fantus (1874–1940), who developed a blood preservation laboratory in Chicago and called it 'The Cook County Hospital Blood Bank', thereby inventing the term 'blood bank'), the Spanish Civil War, in which civilian casualties were prominent, provided the backdrop for the development of a modern blood transfusion service.

Durán-Jordà (Figure 2.7), whose personality was totally different from Bethune's, had established a blood bank in Barcelona prior to Bethune's work in Madrid. In an article in *The Lancet*, he made only tangential reference to the use of blood transfusion in war, even though his designation was 'Late Chief of

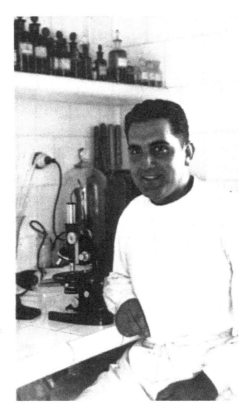

Fig. 2.7 A photograph of Frederick Durán-Jordà.

Reproduced with kind permission from Dr Joan Grifols. Copyright © Joan Grifols.

Blood-Transfusion Service of the Spanish Republican Army' (22). He also made no reference to Bethune in the article, although they apparently had an amicable meeting.

World War II and blood transfusion

War can be an important stimulus to the development of new strategies in medical practice, and World War II proved to be no exception. A key figure around this time was another Bethune-like character, Janet Vaughan, a cousin of Virginia Wolf. Vaughan graduated from Oxford University and conducted research in the Rockefeller Institute at Harvard University before writing a textbook on blood chemistry. She subsequently joined the Royal Postgraduate Medical School in the Hammersmith Hospital, London. In anticipation of war with Germany, she, with others, reviewed the use of stored blood. Interestingly, she failed to mention Bethune's contribution, in spite of the fact that she held similar views on the connection between poverty and disease, was a member of the Communist Party for a short time, and was also friendly with Durán-Jordà. On behalf of the Medical Research Council, she invited Durán-Jordà to England in 1938. He continued to practice haematology there but died prematurely of leukaemia in 1953.

Vaughan, like Bethune, did not suffer authority well but she managed to get agreement from the Medical Research Council and subsequently from the Department of Health in the United Kingdom to establish blood donor centres in London. The first test of her strategy was Dunkirk, and all the evidence suggests that the blood transfusion service saved many lives. During the Blitz, the service once again proved itself and led indirectly to acceptance by the British of stabilizing wounded soldiers with blood transfusion before evacuation. This procedure remains standard practice today.

World War II also stimulated many developments in logistics and science. Scientists, in particular John Elliot in the Rowan Hospital in North Carolina, contributed to the development of a method for separating plasma (the liquid component of blood) from red blood cells. He convinced the authorities that plasma could be shipped to Britain, where it would help treat war casualties in Europe. But even that initiative was hampered by ignorance and prejudice. Charles Drew, an African-American physician, directed the campaign 'Plasma for Britain' but had to battle against racial prejudice to try to prevent the Red Cross from marking blood taken from black Americans so that it would not be transfused into white soldiers. Unfortunately, Drew's campaign failed and he resigned, dying in a car crash at the age of 45.

Besides the logistics, the major problem with plasma was the frequency of contamination with bacteria. A number of scientists and pharmaceutical companies started experimenting with freeze-dried plasma, which could be reconstituted with water. Edwin J. Cohn, a chemist at Harvard University, is an important figure in the development of techniques which are still in use. By adding alcohol to plasma and by varying alcohol concentration, temperature, and centrifuge speeds, he produced a small volume of white powder, which was mostly albumin. He believed this powder would be stable for long periods and could be used to treat shock and blood loss. Cohn's theory was put to the test after the Japanese attack on Pearl Harbor. Albumin proved to be an excellent treatment for shock and burns. However, there was a further problem: albumin had to be reconstituted with water, a time-consuming process with the potential to introduce infection. To address this issue, albumin was packaged in liquid form. During World War II, hundreds of thousands of units of plasma and albumin were transfused, and innumerable lives thereby saved.

While there were many successes, there were also mistakes, particularly in relation to organization and management. A good example, described by Douglas Starr in his book *Blood: An Epic History of Medicine and Commerce* (18), was when thousands of units of blood were transported by air from the United States for use in the Pacific campaign, while the corresponding paperwork was sent by surface mail. The result was that many units of blood were not handled properly and deteriorated before they could be transfused. Blood transfusion, as Bogdanov had remarked earlier, requires good organization as well as scientific endeavour.

With the ending of World War II, the interest in large-scale national blood banking declined, especially in the United States. Once again, Cohn entered the picture, suggesting that blood should always be divided into its component parts after collection so that it could be used more efficiently. However ignorance, prejudice, and fear persisted. And it may seem difficult now for us to believe that such prejudice existed in medical practice such a short time ago. For example, it was illegal in some states until the 1950s to give blood from a black donor to a white recipient without the express permission of the recipient.

The plastic bag: Did it change transfusion medicine?

From the perspective of blood transfusion, the development of a robust plastic bag had many advantages over the glass bottles that had previously been used. Plastic was light, flexible, and easy to transport. The use of plastic bags for blood transfusion became a reality in the early 1950s. Carl W. Walter, a surgeon in the Peter Bent Brigham Hospital at Harvard Medical School, with his colleague William Murphy Jr, designed the first polythene blood collection bag, which had two plastic tubes: one to give blood to the recipient, and the other to collect blood from the donor (23). This flexible plastic bag was used for the first time during the Korean War in the early 1950s, when a lot of experience was gained with its use in transfusion to wounded soldiers (Figure 2.8). So yet again, war became a major stimulus to development; but there were also many technical problems to be overcome before plastic bags were to be commonly used for storing and transfusing blood. Like many developments, prejudice played a role, so that it was not until the mid-1970s that plastic bags were routinely used in the United Kingdom for blood storage and transfusion.

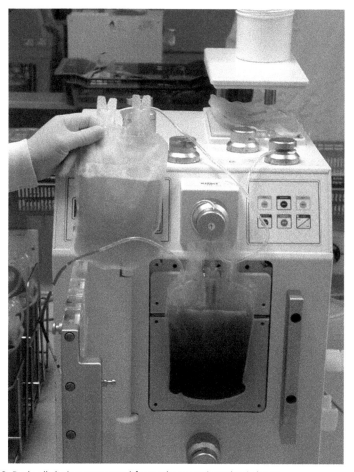

Fig. 2.8 Red cells being separated from plasma using plastic bags.

Reproduced from McCann S, Foà R, Smith O, and Conneally E., *Haematology: Clinical Cases Uncovered*, Second Edition, Wiley/Blackwell, Oxford, UK, Copyright © 2009, with permission from John Wiley and Sons Ltd.

The US government hired Murphy as a consultant during the Korean War, when he performed many blood transfusions using the plastic bag at the front lines. Apart from ease of transport, the development of sealed bags allowed the transfusion of blood under pressure. In other words blood could be transfused quickly, and this development was life-saving for many. However, when Walters wrote a review on transfusion and the plastic bag in 1984, he never mentioned Murphy (24)! Here again, people are left out of the canon for reasons that are not always clear.

Blood substitutes have never become a reality, and today we still rely on the altruistic gift of human donors to allow us to carry out sophisticated surgical and medical treatments. For thousands of years, blood was believed to contain something special such as memory or soul. Relatively recently the life-saving potential of blood transfusion has been realized. War was a major force in the development of the organization of blood supplies and stimulated new technologies. Future research will aim at providing universal donors, perhaps by stripping antigens from the surface of red cells. Nonetheless, the provision of 'artificial blood' still seems a long way off.

References

1 **Riches J.** The Bible: A Very Short Introduction. London, Oxford University Press, 2000.

2 **Díaz B.** The Conquest of New Spain. Translated with an Introduction by J. M. Cohen. Penguin Books, London, 1963.

3 **Harvey W.** De Motu Cordis. William Fitzer, Frankfurt, 1628.

4 **Lower R.** The method observed in transfusing the bloud out of one animal into another. Philosophical Transactions of the Royal Society of London. Series B. Biological Sciences **1** (10): 353–8. 1666.

5 **Boyle R.** Tryals proposed by Mr. Boyle to Dr. Lower, to be made by him, for the improvement of transfusing blood out of one live animal into another. Philosophical Transactions of the Royal Society of London. Series B. Biological Sciences **1** (22): 385–8. 1666.

6 **Coga A.** An account of the experiment of transfusion, practised upon a man in London. Philosophical Transactions of the Royal Society London. Series B. Biological Sciences **2** (30): 557–9. 1667.

7 **Tucker H.** Blood Work: A Tale of Medicine and Murder in the Scientific Revolution. W. W. Norton & Company, New York, NY, 2011.

8 **Blundell J.** Observations on blood transfusion. Lancet **12** (302): 321–4. 1829.

9 **McDonnell R.** Remarks on the Operation of Transfusion and the apparatus for its Performance. The Dublin Quarterly Journal of Medical Science **50** (2): 257–65. 1870.

10 **Rous P, Turner JR.** The preservation of living red blood cells in vitro. I. Methods of preservation. Journal of Experimental Medicine **23** (2): 219–37. 1916.

11 **Rous P, Turner JR.** The preservation of living red blood cells in Vitro. II. The transfusion of kept cells. Journal of Experimental Medicine **23** (2): 239–48. 1916.

12 Stansbury LG, Hess JR. Blood transfusion in World War I: The roles of Lawrence Bruce Robertson and Oswald Hope Robertson in the 'Most Important Medical Advance of the War'. Transfusion Medicine Reviews **23** (3): 232–6. 2009.

13 Pinkerton PH. Canadian surgeons and the introduction of blood transfusion in war surgery. Transfusion Medicine Reviews **22** (1): 77–86. 2008.

14 Editorial. The transfusion of blood. British Medical Journal **2**: 773–4. 1907.

15 Robertson LB. The transfusion of whole blood. A suggestion for its more frequent employment in war surgery. British Medical Journal **2**: 38–40. 1916.

16 Pinkerton PH. Canadian surgeons and the introduction of blood transfusion in war surgery. Transfusion Medicine Reviews **22** (1): 77–86. 2008.

17 Keynes GL. Blood Transfusion. J. Wright, London, 1922.

18 Starr D. Blood: An Epic History of Medicine and Commerce. Quill, New York, NY, 2000.

19 Allan T, Gordon S. The Scalpel and the Sword: The Story of Dr Norman Bethune. Introduction by Julie Allan, Dr. Norman Allan and Susan Ostrovsky. Dundurn Press, Toronto, 2009. (Originally published by McClelland & Stewart, 1952.)

20 Bethune D. Personal communication. 2014.

21 Hannat L. The Politics of Passion: Norman Bethune's Writing and Art. University of Toronto Press, Toronto, 2000.

22 Durán-Jordà F. The Barcelona blood-transfusion service. Lancet **233** (6031): 773–5. 1939.

23 Walter CW, Murphy PW Jr. A closed gravity technique for the preservation of whole blood in ACD solution utilizing plastic equipment. Surgery Gynecology and Obstetrics Archives **94** (6): 687–92. 1972.

24 Walter CW. Invention and development of the blood bag. Vox Sanguinis **47** (4): 318–24. 1984.

Chapter 3

From a dream to a nightmare
HIV, haemophilia, and AIDS

Blood clotting

The mechanism of blood clotting has puzzled and interested doctors and scientists alike since the earliest days. Hippocrates (460–370 BC) and Aristotle (384–322 BC) among others thought that blood was alive inside the body and died when in contact with air (1). It was also believed that cooling blood was the essential mechanism underlying clotting. Galen (130–200) supported the theory of cooling and also believed that blood decayed after leaving the body (1). Much later, William Harvey suggested that there was fibrous mucus in the blood which contributed to blood clotting (1).

We now understand a great deal about the blood clotting process: the biochemical sequence that results in the formation of a life-saving clot. In a healthy state, the final pathway of blood clotting is the generation of thrombin, which exists for a few seconds in the bloodstream. It converts soluble fibrinogen into insoluble fibrin, which interacts with red cells and begins to form a blood clot. Platelets in blood contribute to stabilizing clot formation. In humans, the process of forming a blood clot is usually started by injury to a blood vessel. In a healthy individual, blood clotting is an orderly and self-contained process. The clot is eventually broken down, so that the damaged area is repaired. However, inherited deficiencies in the clotting system can have disastrous effects and sometimes a major influence on history. Figures 3.1 and 3.2 show the current understanding of the coagulation pathway.

Haemophilia: The early days

A bleeding disorder that affected males but transmitted by females has been known since biblical times. *The Salem Gazette*, a weekly newspaper in Massachusetts still in existence, published an obituary in 1791, 'The Earliest Record of Hemophilia in America', reported that Isaac Zoll, a son of Henry Zoll who had come to America from Germany, died of blood loss following an accident with an axe (2). The bleeding could not be stopped, and five of his brothers had died in a similar fashion. The father of the six brothers had married twice and had

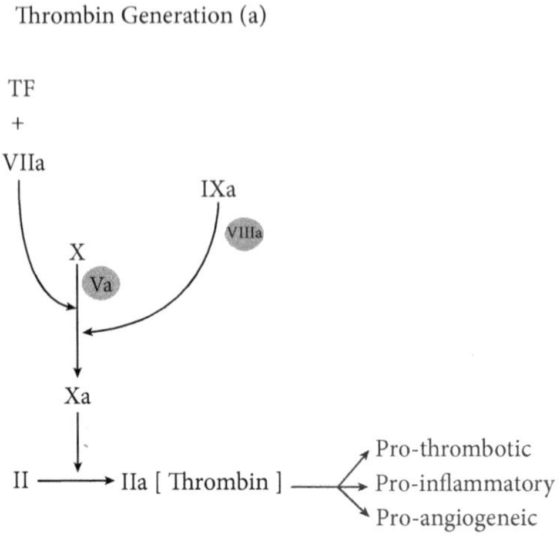

Thrombin Generation (a)

Fig. 3.1 Blood coagulation is initiated when tissue factor (TF), expressed after an injury to the cell wall (e.g. endothelial, monocytic cells), is exposed to Factor VIIa in the bloodstream. The TF-VIIa complex in turn activates Factor IX to Factor IXa, and Factor X to Factor Xa. Factor Xa with its cofactor Factor VIIIa also activates Factor X to Factor Xa (amplification phase). Factor Xa with Factor V activates prothrombin to thrombin, which in turn converts soluble fibrinogen to insoluble fibrin.

Reproduced from McCann S, Foà R, Smith O, and Conneally E., Haematology: Clinical Cases Uncovered, Second Edition, Wiley/Blackwell, Oxford, UK, Copyright © 2009, with permission from John Wiley and Sons Ltd.

several children with each wife. Yet the all the brothers who died had been from the same mother. This crucial observation suggested that the abnormal bleeding tendency was transmitted through the mother. A couple of years later, C. W. H. Consbruch provided the first written description of haemophilia (3). John Conrad Otto (1774–1844), in Pennsylvania, delved deeper into this strange affliction, publishing an account in 1803 of the Smith family in *The Medical Repository*. He described how only the male lines suffered from this 'hemorrhagic disposition', noting that not all males in a family were afflicted. He observed that the mother transmitted the disease to her descendants (4). Maxwell Wintrobe, in his book *Blood, Pure and Eloquent* claimed that Otto was probably the first person to use the term 'bleeder' in his description of the affected males in this family (2). Otto went on to become a famous physician in America and was appointed physician and clinical lecturer of the Pennsylvanian Hospital in 1813.

There is some dispute as to who was the originator of the term 'haemophilia' (2). In 1828 Frederick Hopff (1778–1851), at the University of Zurich, used the term; however, he was a student of Johann Schönlein (1793–1864), who may

Natural Anticoagulant Mechanism (b)

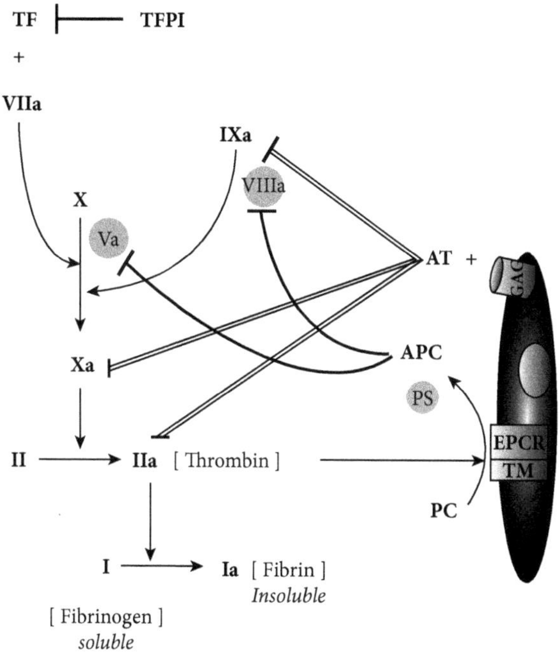

Fig. 3.2 The initiation phase of coagulation is controlled by inhibiting the complex of the tissue factor (TF), Factor VIIa, and Factor Xa by tissue factor pathway inhibitor (TFPI). The amplification phase of coagulation is blocked by the Protein C pathway. Protein C (PC) is activated by a complex of thrombin, thrombomodulin (TM), and endothelial Protein C receptor (EPCR) to form activated Protein C (APC), which in association with Protein S (PS) inactivates Factor Va and Factor VIIa. The thrombin formed in the propagation phase is controlled by antithrombin (AT).

have been the originator of the term. The fact that there was no agreement on how to make a diagnosis inevitably led to a difference of opinion on treatment. Careful history taking could frequently lead to the correct diagnosis, which of course can now be confirmed by appropriate tests.

Attempts at the treatment of haemophilia

In spite of a lack of understanding of the basic defect in bleeding disorders, doctors tried to treat sufferers. For example, in 1840 Samuel Lane encountered bleeding in a young boy following surgery for a squint. From an account published in *The Lancet* the same year, it is evident that neither the surgeon nor his assistants took a full history from the patient or his mother prior to the operation (5). If they had done so, they would have heard evidence of previous bleeding episodes. In order to stop the bleeding, Lane had two major problems to overcome. Firstly, blood groups were unknown at the time and therefore it was pure luck that both donor and patient shared the same blood group. Secondly, the problem of blood clotting during transfusion had not yet been resolved. Lane recorded that only about 150 ml were transfused and the result was dramatic. The bleeding stopped and the patient sat up and had a glass of wine and water. He made a full recovery and his squint was corrected. Whatever the explanation, the transfusion was effective in stopping the bleeding. As the boy received 'whole blood', he would therefore have received plasma at the same time. He probably had von Willebrand disease, not haemophilia.

Royalty and haemophilia

Although Talmudic, and subsequently Arab scholars, had previously delineated the gender-linked nature of severe bleeding disorders (2), our present understanding of how the condition is passed from generation to generation was partly clarified by observing the lives of Europe's royal families. In 1853 Queen Victoria of England gave birth to her eighth child, Leopold, who had haemophilia, despite having previously had three healthy male children. Because it was so common for members of royal families to intermarry, it is easy to trace the condition through the families of Queen Victoria's daughters.

In over 70% of cases of haemophilia, the defective gene is passed from generation to generation. In 30%, however, the disease may appear spontaneously. Because there was no family history of haemophilia on Queen Victoria's side, it is possible that she had a spontaneous mutation which caused haemophilia in her descendants or, as Potts and Potts suggested, she may have been illegitimate (6). If a female carrier has a child, there are four possibilities. The woman may give birth to an unaffected male, a male with haemophilia, an unaffected female, or a female carrier. Therefore, a boy with haemophilia may have an unaffected sister, or his sister may be a carrier (Figures 3.3, 3.4).

Queen Victoria's family provides an example. Her four daughters gave birth to haemophiliac boys, so that clearly the girls were obligate carriers. In other words, they passed on the defective gene on their X chromosome. Haemophilia was thus introduced into both the Spanish and Russian royal families. Although it had been known for centuries that this disorder occurred in males and was transmitted by females, the precise nature of the bleeding defect remained

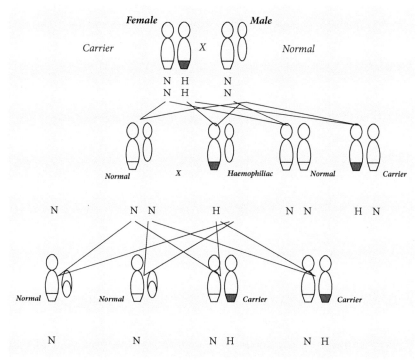

Fig. 3.3 The genetics of haemophilia. Three chromosomes are shown: a normal X chromosome (tip of long arm unshaded), an X chromosome bearing a mutant Factor VIII gene (tip of long arm shaded), and a normal Y chromosome. A female carrier with a normal partner has four possibilities with equal frequency: a normal son, a haemophiliac son, a normal daughter, and a carrier daughter. A haemophiliac male has only two possibilities: a carrier daughter or a normal son; H, haemophiliac; N, normal.

contentious until the late 1930s when the deficient clotting factor, Factor VIII, was determined (2, 7).

Breaking the mould of accepted wisdom is often difficult and, as Oscar Ratnoff pointed out (2), an abstract which began to unravel the immunological and clotting properties of Factor VIII, written by Jacob Shanberge and Ira Gore, was rejected by the Central Society for Clinical Research. Ten years later, two types of haemophilia were delineated: Factor VIII deficiency and Factor IX deficiency. Unravelling the clotting defect led to the development of effective treatment.

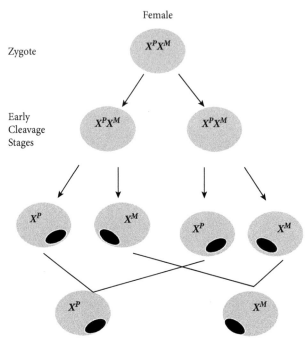

Fig. 3.4 The phenomenon of lyonization. Lyonization (after Mary Lyon, an English geneticist who published her 'random X-inactivation' theory while working at the Medical Research Council laboratory in Harwell, UK) is the name given to inactivation of one member of a pair of X chromosomes in every female cell. It occurs in all somatic cells of the female embryo on the sixteenth day after fertilization, when the embryo is composed of around 5000 cells. For any somatic cell, the choice is whether the paternal (X^p) or the maternal (X^m) X chromosome is inactivated, and this choice is random (the inactive X is shown as a dark mass). Hence, normal females are mosaics with a mixture of X^p and X^m. Because it is a random inactivation, the relative proportions of gene: protein expression vary from female to female. This fact accounts for the variable expression of X-linked recessive traits in heterozygous females.

Reproduced from McCann S, Foà R, Smith O, and Conneally E., Haematology: Clinical Cases Uncovered, Second Edition, Wiley/Blackwell, Oxford, UK, Copyright © 2009, with permission from John Wiley and Sons Ltd.

In the late 1950s and 1960s, the only treatment for a patient with haemophilia was to transfuse frozen plasma from normal donors to supply the missing clotting factors. However, this procedure required large volumes of plasma, and children had to be admitted to hospital, a situation that can cause major family upheavals. A very important breakthrough in the treatment of haemophilia came in 1964 when the scientist Judith Poole made a major discovery: when plasma was rapidly frozen and then slowly thawed, it formed a precipitate, termed 'cryoprecipitate', which contained a large amount of Factor VIII, the anti-haemophilic factor. With administration of cryoprecipitate, surgery in haemophiliacs became safe. The other interesting discovery was that, because haemophilia is an X-linked disease, the phenomenon of X-inactivation means that carriers could have variable levels of Factor VIII (8).

Prophylaxis

Although Inga Mariehad Nilsson first suggested in 1960 in Sweden that children with haemophilia should be given cryoprecipitate regularly to prevent bleeding, prophylaxis did not become widespread until Factor VIII concentrates became available in the late 1960s (9). In most cases, these concentrates were manufactured by commercial pharmaceutical companies, and the patient or a family member administered the concentrate, which was stored in a home freezer. Children with haemophilia were thus able to take part in sports and live a life that was more normal than what had previously been possible.

Hepatitis caused by prophylaxis

However, other problems arose, as treatment with Factor VIII concentrates was sometimes followed by jaundice or abnormal liver blood tests. Subsequently, it was shown that the hepatitis B virus was transmitted via Factor VIII concentrates (10). In 1981 vaccination against hepatitis B was recommended to prevent infection but, in spite of vaccination, a number of recipients of Factor VIII concentrate developed jaundice and abnormal liver blood tests, even though the concentrates were heat-treated to inactivate virus (11). This condition was termed 'non-A, non-B hepatitis'. Most doctors and their patients assumed that non-A, non-B hepatitis, or 'infectious hepatitis', as it was called, was due to an unidentified virus and was a mild, self-limiting illness.

The dark clouds of GRID

However, this so-called mild infection was the harbinger of a deadly disease. In 1981, in the United States, a number of gay men developed infections, including toxoplasmosis, pneumonia caused by pneumocystis carinii, and a very rare skin tumour, Kaposi's sarcoma. Initially, it was believed that this disease was limited to gay men and was called GRID, for 'gay-related immune deficiency syndrome' (12). The US government, under the presidency of Ronald Reagan, declined to provide funding to the Centers for Disease Control and Prevention (CDC) for research into GRID, presumably because the disease had only been reported in gay men (13). By 1982 it became clear that patients with haemophilia were subject to similar infections, and the illness was re-named 'acquired immune deficiency syndrome' (AIDS) (14). In patients af-fected with AIDS, T-lymphocyte numbers were markedly reduced, especially the number of CD4 cells. In 1982 it was also suspected that AIDS could be transmitted by the transfusion of blood or platelets. The aetiological agent was still unidentified but an infectious agent was suspected: 'The etiology of AIDS remains unknown, but its reported occurrence among homosexual men, intravenous drug abusers, and persons with haemophilia A suggests it may be caused by an infectious agent transmitted sexually or through exposure to blood or blood products.' (15).

Could a virus cause GRID?

Why were people with haemophilia getting this disease and why were their im-mune systems so badly damaged? Bruce Evatt at the CDC suggested that a virus was the cause of AIDS and that it was being spread through blood transfusions and Factor VIII concentrates. He conveyed his concerns to the CDC, the Na-tional Institutes of Health, the Federal Drugs Authority, and the National Haemophilia Foundation (16). Since thousands of units of plasma were pooled to make concentrate, blood from one individual with the AIDS virus could con-taminate the entire pool, so that all the vials of concentrate made from the con-taminated pool could become infectious and transmit AIDS.

Following publication of the CDC report in 1982, a public outcry ensued (15). Blood banks refused to take blood from gay male donors, to try to reduce the risk of spreading the infection by blood transfusion. By the mid-1980s, a state of hysteria, reminiscent of that during the years of the medieval plague, had developed among the public, medical, and allied professions. Patients ad-mitted to hospital with haemophilia had their clothes burned, and many hos-pitals tried to cover up the diagnosis of AIDS in haemophiliac patients. The bodies of patients who died of AIDS, including those with haemophilia, were encased in special body bags, and relatives were often refused permission to view them. Pathologists refused to carry out post-mortem examinations on pa-tients with AIDS. Some hospitals even refused to treat AIDS patients. The late William F. Buckley, a well-known American Republican commentator, was quoted as proposing that everybody with AIDS should have a tattoo on their forearm and buttocks stating: 'Our society is generally threatened' (17).

Nonetheless, national and commercial concerns took precedence over patient safety: blood donations which were not tested for HIV continued to be collected and used. In many countries, both infected individuals and haemophilia societies later brought court cases against state agencies and pharmaceutical companies, but these were usually unsuccessful, or the damages awarded were minor. But the public's perception of the safety of blood and blood products had changed forever.

Interestingly, early on, in the absence of a blood test for AIDS, it was found that the incidence of transmission of AIDS by blood transfusion began to decrease when donor selection was undertaken by blood banks and when testing for the hepatitis B core antigen (anti-HBc) as a surrogate marker for AIDS was introduced into blood banks. However, many blood and plasma collection agencies rejected anti-HBc testing which, according to the Institute of Medicine, probably would have reduced the number of individuals infected with HIV through blood and blood products (18). The other approach was through requesting the details of the sexual behaviour of potential donors. Initially, there was resistance to such intrusive questioning of blood and plasma donors, for fear of scaring them away (19). More recently, however, in the interest of public health, questionnaires have become unapologetically intrusive (see Box 3.1).

Were the media a help or a hindrance at this time? It is difficult to be sure. The public must be informed of health hazards, but scare tactics can make a bad situation worse. The number of blood donors decreased, although blood banks

Box 3.1 Example of questions given to all potential blood, plasma, and platelet donors

This is a typical example of a questionnaire of potential blood donors.

1 Are you giving bloods to be tested for HIV, AIDS or hepatitis?
2 Have you ever injected or been injected with non-prescription drugs— even once or a long time ago? This includes bodybuilding drugs.
3 If you are a male, have you ever had oral or anal sex with another male— even if a condom or other protection was used?
4 Have you ever received money or drugs for sex?
5 Do you or your partner have HIV/AIDS?
6 Do you or your partner or close household contacts have hepatitis B or C?

If the answer to any of the above is YES, or if you are in any doubt, you must indicate YES, and not donate.

Reproduced from the Irish Blood Transfusion Service questionnaire, under the Re-use of Public Sector Information Regulations 2005 (SI 279 of 2005), https://www.giveblood.ie/Re-use_of_Public_Sector_Information/. Copyright © 2015 Irish Blood Transfusion Service.

were trying to improve the safety of blood transfusion. People began to believe that a healthy donor could contract AIDS by giving blood.

The pharmaceutical industry

The results of research were not heeded or acted upon for many years because the findings threatened corporate interests. A potential conflict arose between blood banks and the pharmaceutical industry because the industry needed donations to manufacture Factor VIII concentrates, and blood banks needed to insist on new questionnaires and screening procedures. Many pharmaceutical companies rejected the claim of a direct link between the use of Factor VIII concentrates and the transmission of AIDS. Thus, a state of denial among both blood banks and pharmaceutical companies evolved, as both looked upon the catastrophe of contaminated blood and factor concentrates as an unimaginable disaster. When the pharmaceutical company Cutter was forced to destroy 64,000 vials of Factor VIII concentrate because of the possibility of transmitting AIDS, their spokesman Bud Modersbach argued that Cutter were doing this in the absence of evidence that AIDS could be transmitted via Factor VIII concentrates and that they were taking this action to show the public that every precaution was being taken.

Throughout 1983 and 1984, the story continued to reveal a combination of human frailty, scientific jealousy, and the ability of governments and state agencies to put commercial concerns before patient safety. In 1992 Michael Garretta, the former head of France's national centre for blood transfusion, and his associate, Jean-Pierre Allain, who was the former head of research at the same institute, received prison sentences and hefty fines.

Could more have been done?

Could more have been done to stop the transmission of AIDS via blood transfusion and contaminated blood products? Perhaps. Although the cause of AIDS had not been identified in the early years of the AIDS crisis, most people working in the field at that time believed that it was transmitted by an unidentified virus. Identification of the virus was therefore important, because it could lead to a test which would immediately screen and eliminate infected donors. But were there other ways that could have been used to stop the transmission of AIDS via blood products? In spite of all the media speculation and fear in the community, a simple method of inactivating viruses in Factor VIII concentrates was ignored. Ten years before the first AIDS case had been diagnosed, Edward Shanbrom, in the United States, discovered that the introduction of a detergent which broke up the fat coating around a virus could make the virus non-infectious. He received a patent for this method and tried without success to persuade a number of pharmaceutical manufacturers to use it (20). Another method which could successfully destroy some viruses was heat treatment. Even after the FDA approved heat treatment of blood products, it is extraordinary to think that many Factor VIII concentrates continued to be manufactured in the old way for at least another year (19).

HIV and blood transfusion

In the early 1980s, the search for the causative virus intensified. In the competitive arena of scientific research, Luc Montagnier and colleagues in 1983 at the Institut Pasteur in Paris discovered the virus that caused AIDS and called it LAV (lymphadenopathy-associated virus). It was recovered from a swollen lymph gland from a patient with AIDS; however, it was not yet clear that this virus caused AIDS. Montagnier and his team sent samples to Robert Gallo at the National Institutes of Health in Washington, where the Gallo team then claimed to have discovered a new virus they called HTLV-III. Both viruses were, however, identical. A bitter French–US row ensued, with claims and counter-claims, but justice prevailed in 2008 when Montagnier and his colleague Françoise Barré-Sinoussi, shared the Nobel Prize for Medicine or Physiology for their discovery of the HIV (AIDS) virus (Figure 3.5).

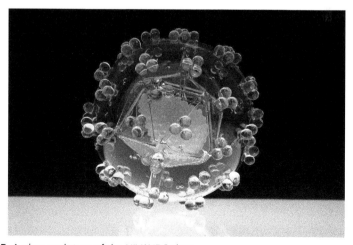

Fig. 3.5 A glass sculpture of the HIV/AIDS virus.

Photograph by Luke Jerram. Reproduced by kind permission of the artist, Luke Jerram. Copyright © 2015 Luke Jerram.

Once the virus was identified, the test for its presence, or antibodies to it, became the next objective. With the HIV virus, although antibodies against it are not protective, they still serve as a marker of infection. Therefore, a simple, cheap, and rapid test for the presence of the anti-HIV antibody was possible. However, although such a test was urgently required, once again nationalism played a part, and the antibody screening test developed by Abbott in the United States was not introduced into France for another year.

While undoubtedly we have made advances in our understanding of transmission of infectious diseases via blood transfusion, the transfusion of a biological fluid from one person to another will always be accompanied by a degree of uncertainty and risk. While plasma and Factor VIII concentrates can be treated to kill viruses such as HIV, such treatments damage red cells and therefore cannot be used to make blood transfusions safe. Thus, careful screening of blood donors remains of paramount importance. The other issue is the so-called window period between infection with HIV and the development of antibodies against it, so that it may be weeks before an individual who has contracted HIV infection will test positive for anti-HIV antibodies. A new assay which can detect the virus via nucleic acid testing has been developed but is extremely expensive. In the meantime, intrusive questionnaires and antibody testing has reduced the incidence of transmission of the HIV virus via blood transfusion to very low levels— even to zero, in some countries—by the mid-1990s. In 2013 a number of blood transfusion services began to allow gay men to act as blood donors.

Recombinant technology enables the manufacture of large volumes of novel proteins synthesized in a laboratory. The first example of the successful large-scale manufacture of a synthetic protein was the production of recombinant insulin. In the case of haemophilia, synthetic Factor VIII is available but is very expensive, and in many countries its use is limited to newly diagnosed patients.

The spread of HIV infection by both hetero- and homosexual contact is, however, a global issue. Donald G. McNeil Jr, writing in *The International Herald Tribune* in 2010 pointed out that, in the early 2000s, hopes began to rise for a cure for AIDS, with the advent of cheap antiretroviral drugs. Although there was no HIV vaccine, a scheme for the use of anti-AIDS drugs was initiated by Kofi Annan, the Secretary General of the United Nations at that time, and the US president, George W. Bush, through the Global Fund. Unfortunately, with the recent worldwide economic downturn, the supply of cheap anti-AIDS drugs has dwindled. There has also been a shift in political thinking linked to the universal economic downturn. Many donor organizations have therefore decided to refocus aid to potentially eradicable diseases like malaria, diarrhoeal diseases, tetanus, and measles.

Reflecting on the tragic story of HIV/AIDS and the role of blood and blood product transfusion, it is clear that the outcome reflects the huge complexity of the relationship between medicine, society, politics, and industry. The philosophy behind blood transfusion has been influenced to a large extent by Richard Titmuss's book *The Gift Relationship*. (21). He extols an altruistic attitude to blood transfusion that eschews paid donors. As a sociologist, Titmuss had a profound effect on the politics of blood transfusion services in the United Kingdom and the United States. In an article by Kieran Healy in 1999, the attitudes advanced by Titmuss are criticized, and the fact that volunteer donors were as responsible for spreading HIV/AIDS as paid donors were is highlighted (22). Healy claims that 'Titmuss's system ended up selecting the wrong people in much the same way the previous market arrangement (paid donors) had selected the wrong people: by accident'. Whatever your view about paid versus altruistic donors, the possibility of disasters occurring will always exist.

Congenital bleeding disorders

We now know that haemophilia is caused by mutations in the genes for Factor VIII or Factor IX, both of which are located on the X chromosome, and that haemophilia A is almost ten times as common as haemophilia B. Although over 200 mutations have been identified, almost 50% of haemophilia A cases are caused by an inversion of Intron 22, a finding which simplifies the diagnosis and genetic counselling. Because Alexis, the son of the Czar and Czarina of Russia, had severe haemophilia, it was assumed until recently that he suffered from haemophilia A, that is, Factor VIII deficiency. However, the discovery in 2007 of a tomb containing the Czar's family revealed, using genetic investigations, that Alexis suffered from severe haemophilia B, and not A as was generally assumed (23).

Not all congenital blood clotting factor deficiencies are associated with bleeding. Some are found in specific racial groups. A good example is Factor XII deficiency. Although patients with Factor XII deficiency have an increased time of coagulation (as determined by the activated partial thromboplastin time test), they do not bleed excessively. In fact, the first patient described with Factor XII deficiency died from a pulmonary embolus (24). Deficiencies in all other coagulation factors have been described but are rare. Factor XI deficiency, found almost exclusively in Ashkenazi Jews, can cause serious bleeding but only if the level of the deficient factor falls below 1%.

The most common disorder, and some are reluctant to call it a disease, is von Willebrand disease. This condition is due to a deficiency of von Willebrand factor, a multimeric plasma protein that facilitates platelet adhesion to injured blood vessels and protects Factor VIII from rapid proteolytic degradation. The disease was first described by a Finnish doctor, Erik Adolf von Willebrand, in 1926 (25). A mild-mannered and humble man, he described the bleeding disorder in a family on the Åland Islands. The molecular basis of the disease is due to either a partial deficiency in the synthesis of von Willebrand factor or a functional abnormality in the protein. Levels of von Willebrand factor are linked to blood groups. People with Group O blood tend to have lower levels of the factor than those with Group AB blood. Women exhibit more symptoms of bleeding than men, and type 1 von Willebrand disease probably contributes to menorrhagia. There are a number of types of von Willebrand disease, some of which are associated with severe platelet-type bleeding (easy bruising and bleeding from mucosal surfaces); but the commonest type is type 1 von Willebrand disease. According to J. Evan Saddler, however, type 1 von Willebrand disease is very difficult to diagnose, and many people with the diagnosis do not bleed abnormally (26). If treatment for type 1 von Willebrand disease is required, DDAVP (desmopressin) is effective, as it stimulates the release of von Willebrand factor from Weibel–Palade bodies in endothelial cells. It can be given intranasally or intravenously. Anti-fibrinolytic agents such as tranexamic acid are also useful. However, Sadler points out that there is a poor correlation between bleeding and levels of von Willebrand factor, unless the levels are very low, and recommends 'an empiric epidemiologic approach like that applied to other modest risk factors for disease such as elevated cholesterol and high blood pressure' (26).

Congenital bleeding disorders remain major problems in countries where medical services are not well developed. By contrast new understanding and technology have come to the rescue in developed countries, where effective treatment allows people to lead an almost normal life. One of the greatest challenges, however, in the past few decades has been the complex sociological and medical problem of AIDS/HIV. Although there is now hope that a vaccine will be developed and the disease eradicated, the massive death toll is a reminder that technology cannot solve all problems. This fact was illuminated by a recent conversation with Smbat Dagbashyan in Yerevan, Armenia, when he told me that, in his country, there had only been a single case of HIV/AIDS in a haemophiliac patient because the medical establishment could not afford to purchase concentrates of Factor VIII or Factor IX and had relied instead on the old method of using plasma and cryoprecipitate for treatment (27).

References

1 **Bynum W.** The History of Medicine: A Very Short Introduction. Oxford University Press, Oxford, 2008.
2 **Wintrobe MW, ed.** Blood, Pure and Eloquent. McGraw-Hill, Inc., New York, NY, 1980.

3 **Bulloch W, Fildes P**. Hemophilia, in K. Pearson, ed., Treasury of Human Inheritance. Dulau & Co., London, 1911, pp. 167–354.

4 **Otto JC**. An account of an hemorrhagic disposition existing in certain families. Medical Repository **6**: 1–4. 1803.

5 **Lane S**. Haemorrhagic diathesis: Successful transfusion of blood. Lancet **41** (4): 185–8. 1840.

6 **Potts DM, Potts WTW**. Queen Victoria's Gene: Haemophilia and the Royal Family. Fourth edition. Sutton Publishing, Stroud, 1999.

7 **Patek AJ Jr, Taylor FHL**. Hemophilia II. Some properties of a substance obtained from normal plasma effective in accelerating the clotting of hemophilic blood. Journal of Clinical Investigation **16** (1): 113–24. 1937.

8 **Lyon MF**. Gene action in the X-chromosomes of the mouse (*Mus musculus* L.). Nature **190** (4773): 372–3. 1961.

9 **Nilsson IM, Blombäck M, Blombäck B**. The use of human antihaemophilic globulin (Fraction 1–0) in haemophilia A and in von Willebrand's disease. Acta Haematologica **24** (1–3): 116–23. 1960.

10 **Forbes CD, Lowe GD**, eds, Unresolved Problems in Haemophilia. MTP Press, Lancaster, 1982, pp. 27–37.

11 **Colombo M, Carnelli V, Gazengel C, Mannucci PM, Savidge GF, Schimpf K**. Transmission of non-A, non-B hepatitis by heat-treated Factor VIII concentrates. Lancet **326** (8445) 1–4. 1985.

12 Centers for Disease Control. A cluster of Kaposi's sarcoma and *Pneumocystis carinii* pneumonia among homosexual male residents of Los Angeles and Orange County, California. Morbidity and Mortality Weekly Report **31** (23): 305–7. 1982.

13 **Altman LK**. New homosexual disorder worries health officials. The New York Times. 11 May 1982.

14 **Sepkowitz KA**. AIDS: The first 20 years. New England Journal of Medicine **344** (23): 1764–72. 2001.

15 Morbidity and Mortality Weekly Reports. Epidemiologic notes and reports possible transfusion-associated acquired immune deficiency syndrome (AIDS): California. Morbidity and Mortality Weekly Reports **31** (48): 652–4. 1982.

16 **Evatt BL**. The tragic history of AIDS in the hemophilia population 1982–1984. Journal of Thrombosis and Hemostasis **4** (11): 2295–301. 2006.

17 **Buckley WF**. Crucial steps in combating the AIDS epidemic: Identify all the carriers. The New York Times on the Web. 18 Mar 1986. www.nytimes.com/books/00/07/16/specials/buckley-aids.html, 1986.

18 Institute of Medicine. HIV and the Blood Supply: An Analysis of Crisis Decision-making. National Academy Press, Washington, DC, 1995.

19 **Sullivan R**. Blood plasma is withdrawn as AIDS link. The New York Times. 2 Nov 1983.

20 **Starr D**. Blood: An Epic History of Medicine and Commerce. Warner Books, London, 2000. (Originally published by Alfred Knopf, Inc., 1998.)

21 **Titmuss RM**. The Gift Relationship: From Human Blood to Social Policy. George Allen & Unwin, London, 1970.

22 **Healy K**. The emergence of HIV in the U.S. blood supply: Organizations, obligations, and the management of uncertainty. Theory and Society **28** (4): 529–58. 1999.

23 **Lannoy C, Hermans C**. The royal disease: Haemophilia A or B? A haematological mystery is finally solved. Haemophilia **16** (6): 343–7. 2010.

24 **Ratnoff, O**. Personal communication. 1975.

25 **Willebrand EA von**. Hereditary pseudohaemophilia. Haemophilia **5** (3): 223–31. 1999.

26 **Sadler JE**. Von Willebrand disease type 1: A diagnosis in search of a disease. Blood **101** (6): 2089–93. 2003.

27 **Dagbashyan S**. Personal communication. 2015.

Chapter 4

Red blood cells

How they live and how they die

Haemolytic anaemias: Rare but informative

Although haemolytic anaemias are relatively rare conditions, the biochemical unravelling of these disorders has opened a Pandora's box of interesting findings. The understanding of the physiology and pathobiology of cell metabolism and human disease has provided insight which reaches far beyond the frequency of these disorders.

Red blood cells

Red blood cells, also known as erythrocytes, are unique in that they do not contain a nucleus. This fact makes the study of their metabolism a little easier than it is for other cells. Their diameter is 7.0 µm. They have a beautiful bi-concave disc shape which is ideal for deformability, as they must traverse openings which have a very small diameter (e.g. 3.0 µm in the spleen). In the early embryo, they are manufactured in the liver but, in children and adults, the bone marrow is the source of erythrocytes under normal circumstances (Figure 4.1). Erythrocytes contain the protein pigment haemoglobin, which is in solution in the cells and consists of globin chains and iron.

The role of the microscope in haematology

When haematologists refer to the microscope, they mean the compound microscope. The Romans had simple magnifying glasses, but Roger Bacon (1214–94) is credited with first combining lenses (1). Bacon was an English philosopher and lectured at Oxford and Paris. He became a Franciscan friar at the age of 42 years and was a good friend of Pope Clement IV. Following the Pope's death, Bacon was imprisoned for his belief in alchemy (a common belief among scientists) but he eventually returned to Oxford, where he died. He was influenced by the two great Arabic scientists, Ibn Sahl (940–1000), a Jew who converted to Islam in Spain, and Ibn al-Haytham (956–1039). Ibn Sahl was a mathematician and optics engineer and is credited with the first description of the law of refraction. He used it to make curved lenses which had no geometric aberrations.

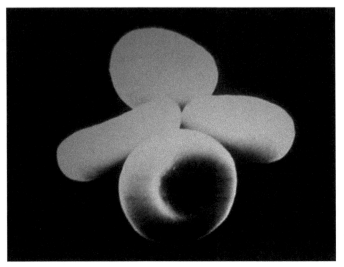

Fig. 4.1 Scanning electron microscope photograph of the author's erythrocytes.

Reproduced by kind permission of Shaun McCann. Copyright © 2015 Shaun McCann.

Credit for the first compound microscope goes to Zacharias Jannsen and his father Hans, both Dutch spectacle makers, around 1590 (2). They put several lenses in a tube and discovered that the object near the end appeared to be greatly magnified. Further developments were made by Anton van Leeuwenhoek (1632–1723) and Robert Hooke (1635–1703). Hooke was a natural philosopher and polymath, like many of his contemporaries. He was a colleague and close friend of Robert Boyle and held the post of curator of experiments at the Royal Society. Although he is best known for his survey and remodelling of London after the Great Fire, he was a keen microscopist, making major contributions to the theory of light refraction.

Who was the first person to recognize the shape of erythrocytes?

Van Leeuwenhoek was not a scientist but a draper who lived in Delft and had an interest in lens making; he developed lenses from tiny spheres of glass. Using these lenses, he was the first to describe bacteria, spermatozoa, and blood flowing through a capillary (Figure 4.2). He made his observations known to the Royal Society rather than in publications and, although he had a tempestuous relationship with the Royal Society, his observations were eventually vindicated. Jan Swammerdam (1637–80) was a biologist who graduated in medicine

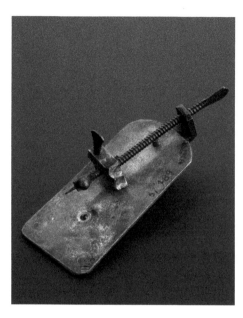

Fig. 4.2 A copy of Van Leeuwenhoek's microscope.

Reproduced from Wellcome Library, London. Image ID: L0057739. Library reference no.: Science Museum A500644. Copyright © 2015 Science Museum, London, Wellcome Images, London, UK.

from the University of Leiden and, following a short spell in France, returned to Leiden, where he carried out his research. He was the first to describe the size and shape of red corpuscles (2). Robert Hooke was the first to use the term 'cell' to describe microorganisms but there is no record of him providing a description of erythrocytes. In the eighteenth century, Gabriel Andral (1779– 1876), a French pathologist, and William Addison (1803–81), an English physician, both described the leukocyte, and Addison deduced that pus cells were leukocytes that had passed through capillaries (2). However, it wasn't until the middle of the nineteenth century that haematology began in earnest. Alfred Donné, a French public health physician, was an enthusiastic microscopist who discovered *Trichomonas vaginalis* in Parisian prostitutes but also discovered blood platelets (3). The credit for the latter discovery is somewhat disputed, as the Italians give the credit for it to Giulio Bizzozero. Donné also developed the photoelectric microscope and held 'workshops' in microscopy, although his discoveries were often met with indifference or hostility by the medical profession. The microscope was considered a source of error, with the images being the result of an artefact. The images are, of course, the result of an artefact but one that is reproducible, thus allowing scientists and doctors to make comparisons and deductions about the aetiology and pathogenesis of disease. The development of staining techniques helped significantly in this regard. Donné was the first to use the daguerreotype to illustrate his microscopic findings.

John Hughes Bennett, the famous English physician and pathologist, studied under Donné while in Paris and said that Donné was 'persevering and enthusiastic'. Although Donné eventually overcame the hostility from the medical profession, he was never accepted as a professor and gave his lectures and demonstrations in a building opposite the medical school, supporting them with his own money. He used the daguerreotype to make illustrations of what he saw with the microscope. The medical profession was slow to adopt this important instrument (4).

The daguerreotype

As for developing a procedure for blood transfusion in the seventeenth century, there was competition between the English and the French to produce photographic images that would not fade. The French chemist and artist Louis-Jacques-Mandé Daguerre (1787–1851) worked with Joseph Niépce (1765–1833), a French inventor in the early nineteenth century. Following Niépce's death in 1833, Daguerre went on to invent a method of developing faint images, although, unfortunately, this method was rather slow. He subsequently developed a technique for 'fixing' the image in a solution of sodium chloride, and in 1837 he produced 'L'Atelier de l'artiste', the first daguerreotype to undergo exposure, development, and fixation. The French Academy of Science announced the invention of the daguerreotype in 1839; later that year, the Englishman William Fox Talbot announced his silver chloride 'sensitive paper' process. Thus was photography born.

The erythrocyte lifespan

Once red cells had been identified, the following philosophical and practical question arose: do red cells live forever and, if not, what is their lifespan? Although every medical student today knows that erythrocytes live in the circulation for 100–120 days (unlike polymorphs, which leave the circulation in a random fashion–sometimes in ≥1 hour), in fact, the lifespan of a red cell was only established fairly recently. Sir John Dacie in Volume 1 of *The Haemolytic Anaemias* says that William Hunter was the first to use the term 'haemolytic', in 1888 (5). In Wintrobe's book *Blood, Pure and Eloquent*, Dacie goes into detail about the experiments which established the erythrocyte lifespan (1). Many of these seminal experiments would not be permitted now because of 'health and safety' or lack of 'Ethical Institutional Board' approval. Premature destruction of red cells (haemolysis) had been clearly described in the nineteenth century by Lucas Dressler (6) but it was well into the twentieth century before the lifespan of the erythrocyte was definitively established. The experiments of Winifred

Ashby (1879–1975) in the Mayo Clinic, involving the transfusion of incompatible red cells and measuring the time to the disappearance of agglutinated cells, predicted a lifespan of around 100 days (7); this finding was later confirmed by studies using ^{32}P-labelled diisopropylfluorophosphonate and radioactive chromium (^{51}Cr) studies (1). Erythrocytes may leave the circulation through blood loss or may be destroyed prematurely in the spleen or within blood vessels. The bone marrow has an innate capacity to increase the production of erythrocytes and, even in the face of premature destruction of erythrocytes, the haemoglobin concentration of the blood may remain within normal limits.

Why erythrocytes leave the circulation after 100–120 days is unknown. However, the fact that they circulate for so long without a nucleus or ribosomes for protein synthesis is remarkable. They are removed from the circulation by macrophages in the spleen, and their contents are reused. This process can actually be harmful, as the reutilization of iron when red cells are prematurely destroyed in the spleen may cause the ill effects of iron overload. Conversely, it is also true that the recycling of iron is very important when it is in short supply.

Haemolysis

Premature destruction of erythrocytes, in the absence of blood loss, is termed haemolysis. If the bone marrow is unable to compensate adequately, anaemia ensues and the condition is called haemolytic anaemia. As we saw in Chapter 1, Pythagoras forbade his followers to ingest fava beans because the beans might cause them to become jaundiced and die (the condition termed 'favism'). The underlying defect in favism is a deficiency in the activity of the enzyme glucose-6-phosphate dehydrogenase (G6PD); this deficiency results in the destruction of red cells because of oxidative stress. However, this mechanism was not understood until the 1950s (8) and required the unravelling of the metabolism of glucose in red cells (Figure 4.3). A deficiency in G6PD activity reduces the amount of NADPH, resulting in a reduction in the amount of glutathione disulfide. Consequently, haemoglobin is degraded and deposited within erythrocytes as Heinz bodies.

In *ASH 50th Anniversary Reviews*, Ernest Beutler makes an extraordinary statement referring to prisoners in the Illinois State Penitentiary at Joliet who were given antimalarial drugs (8-aminoquinolines). He says 'these men were volunteers in the true sense of the word. There was no coercion, and all signed informed consent that spelled out in detail what was to be done . . . The discovery of G6PD deficiency is a clear example of how clinical studies carried out on prisoner volunteers can benefit society and save lives without harm to anyone' (9). He does not mention how many of these men were African Americans, who would

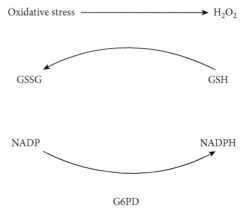

Fig. 4.3 A diagrammatic representation of the hexose monophosphate shunt in red blood cells; G6PD, glucose-6-phosphate dehydrogenase; GSH, glutathione; GSSH, glutathione disulphide.

have had an increased chance of carrying the mutant G6PD enzyme compared to Caucasians of European descent. His claim that these prisoners were true 'volunteers' appears to be somewhat naive, as one cannot imagine that some amelioration of sentence was not available to 'volunteers'. Some prisoners became jaundiced, and subsequent cross-transfusion experiments (which would not be allowed today) demonstrated that the red cells were abnormal in the jaundiced prisoners. This condition was initially known as primaquine sensitivity (10).

Eventually, the mechanisms of haemolysis were worked out, although some animal experiments still question the proposed mechanisms. There are now many known *G6PD* mutations that are associated with altered activity. Mutations of the gene occur in areas where malaria is endemic and in African Americans. As the gene is X-linked, the activity in the putative carrier will be variable because of random X-inactivation, as with Factor VIII in haemophilia carriers. Female carriers will be mosaics; that is, some of their red cells will contain normal G6PD, and others will have the mutant enzyme. The protective effect of G6PD mutations against malaria was investigated by Lucio Luzzatto and colleagues and published in 1969 (11). They showed that G6PD-deficient cells in putative carriers were inherently resistant to malarial infection.

Since then, the G6PD gene has been cloned and the mutations defined: the G6PD A isoform is a result of a substitution of aspartic acid for asparagine, but G6PD A– is not caused by a single mutation but by a number of variants. In spite of all the publications about G6PD deficiency, clinical problems remain (12). Screening tests are now available and should be employed in populations where G6PD deficiency is prevalent and when drugs such as dapsone, primaquine, or nitrofurantoin are prescribed. An enzymopathy has therefore become a public health issue.

Paroxysmal nocturnal haemoglobinuria: From the bedside to the bench

In stark contrast to G6PD deficiency, paroxysmal nocturnal haemoglobinuria is a rare disease, with an incidence of about 5 per million, which has triggered a lot of biochemical investigation and deepened our understanding of the mechanisms of complement activation. Although the disease was probably recognized as early as 1793 (13), Paul Strübing's paper, published in 1882, identified it as a distinct entity (14). It took a considerable amount of time before the genetics and molecular biology of this disease were clarified. In 1939 Thomas Ham published his famous Ham test, also known as the acidified serum lysis test (15), but it took a further 17 years before the alternative complement pathway was incriminated in the haemolysis (16). Shortly before this discovery, the importance of thrombosis as a cause of death in paroxysmal nocturnal haemoglobinuria had been recognized (17). In the mid-1960s, Wendell Rosse and John Dacie demonstrated that erythrocyte populations from patients with paroxysmal nocturnal haemoglobinuria were mosaic and that lysis only occurred in the complement-sensitive population of red cells (18, 19). The Ham test and the sucrose lysis test (20) remained the standard diagnostic tests until flow cytometry replaced them. The flow cytometric profile depended on the understanding of the absence or partial deficiency of the glycosylphosphatidylinositol-anchored proteins on the erythrocyte surface (21) (Figure 4.4). Taroh Kinoshita and colleagues showed that paroxysmal nocturnal haemoglobinuria is a consequence of mutations in the *PIGA* (phosphatidylinositol glycan-class A) gene (13), and Luzzatto points out that over 150 mutations have been elucidated in patients with paroxysmal nocturnal haemoglobinuria (21). The paroxysmal nocturnal haemoglobinuria phenotype is determined by the *PIGA* genotype, and paroxysmal nocturnal haemoglobinuria is an oligoclonal disorder (22).

Treatment of paroxysmal nocturnal haemoglobinuria

Has all this clever biochemistry been translated into effective treatment for paroxysmal nocturnal haemoglobinuria? This story has a happy ending, although there are still some questions and problems to be overcome. If the haemolysis and many of the other clinical manifestations of paroxysmal nocturnal haemoglobinuria are complement mediated, then the development of an anti-complement agent seems appropriate, bearing in mind the importance of complement in the immune system. It also seemed logical to aim at complement component 5 (C5), as thus the early part of the complement cascade would be left intact. Thus, a drug that had been around for some time became a focus for those seeking an effective

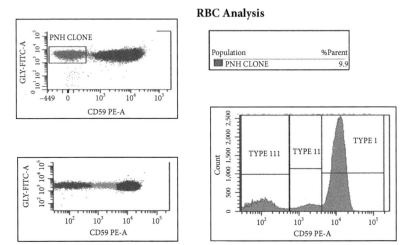

Fig. 4.4 Flow cytometry analysis of red blood cells from two patients with paroxysmal nocturnal haemoglobinuria. The dot plots for the two patients are shown on the left (top plot, Patient A; bottom plot, Patient B). In the plots, three populations of red blood cells can be seen, as characterized by their expression of the membrane protein CD59, which is normally anchored to the cell membrane by glycosylphosphatidylinositol. The cells have been labelled with two markers: glycine tagged with fluorescein isothiocyanate (GLY-FITC-A; labels all red blood cells), and an anti-CD59 antibody tagged with the fluorescent dye phycoerythrin (CD59 PE-A). The population on the left (indicated in the top plot by a box and the label 'PNH CLONE') represents the cells that completely lack CD59; these are termed type III PNH cells and make up 9.9% of the total red blood cell population in Patient A. The population on the right represents cells with normal levels of CD59; these are termed type I PNH cells. In Patient B, a third population (in the middle; indicated in light grey) can be distinguished; this population represents cells that express reduced levels of CD59 (type II PNH cells). The histogram on the right shows the distribution of the three populations in Patient B; RBC, red blood cell.

treatment for paroxysmal nocturnal haemoglobinuria (23). A humanized monoclonal antibody which binds to C5, called eculizumab, had previously been used to treat autoimmune diseases like rheumatoid arthritis, glomerulonephritis, and systemic lupus erythematosus. Although not very effective, it did bind to C5 and thus prevented the formation of the 'membrane attack' complex. Importantly, although life-threatening and fatal meningococcal infections have occurred in patients treated with eculizumab, only one case of meningococcal infection was reported in 700 treated patients. A number of studies showed that, when used in patients with paroxysmal nocturnal haemoglobinuria, eculizumab was associated with a reduction in transfusion requirement, a decrease in thrombotic episodes, an improvement in renal function, and an improvement in quality of life (24, 25) and the drug is licensed in many countries for this indication.

A clinical feature of paroxysmal nocturnal haemoglobinuria which can be very debilitating is dysphagia. Nitric oxide is consumed by free haemoglobin during intravascular haemolysis. Although well recognized in sickle cell anaemia, this mechanism for dysphagia, lethargy, and pulmonary hypertension has only been recognized relatively recently in paroxysmal nocturnal haemoglobinuria (26). However, two major problems remain. Firstly, eculizumab is extremely expensive and, secondly, it is necessary with this drug to have visits every 2 weeks to the clinic for intravenous administration.

The sad fact, as any practising haematologist will tell you, is that there is usually a long gap between the first symptoms and a final diagnosis of paroxysmal nocturnal haemoglobinuria, and many patients are subjected to extensive renal investigations because doctors don't differentiate between haematuria and haemoglobinuria. (In this case, a dip stick test won't help. You need to look down a microscope!)

Rare diseases can teach us a lot but the initiating observation is usually clinical, that is, at the bedside, and from there it takes persistent and well-designed laboratory studies before the pathobiology of the disease is unravelled (at the bench) and hopefully effective treatment developed (back to the bedside).

Spherocytes: Congenital or acquired?

How does a bi-concave disc become a sphere? It does so by reducing the ratio of surface area to volume. This reduction can occur because of a congenital membrane abnormality or if membrane is lost, usually by phagocytosis. Phagocytosis occurs when antibodies or complement are present on the red cell membrane and are removed by macrophages (27, 28). A small amount of red cell membrane is removed at the same time, thus creating a spherocyte. To see a spherocyte requires microscopic examination of a well-made blood film, and to tell an acquired spherocyte from a congenital one requires a Coombs' test. According to Charles Packman (29), the first case of acquired haemolytic anaemia was described by Galen. In his historical review, C. Dreyfus (30) says that Galen treated a slave of Emperor Marcus Aurelius with theriaca following a snake bite as the slave's 'skin turned the colour of a ripe leek'. We don't know the outcome or if the slave had spherocytes, but theriaca elixir is still sold as a total body medicine and contains antioxidants, such as resveratrol, and beta-glucans, among other 'nutrients' and 'minerals'.

Although acquired haemolytic anaemia due to 'cold' antibodies had been described since 1890, the true mechanism was not understood until Robin Coombs was able to demonstrate antibody and/or complement on the surface of the red cell via the direct antiglobulin test (31); this test remains the most important test for antibody-mediated haemolytic anaemia available. Coombs, a veterinarian, is quoted as saying: 'In a flash I could see the globulin antibody on the red cells and these cells should be agglutinated with an antibody to serum globulin, i.e. an antiglobulin. All the thinking had been done' (32). Serendipitously, Muriel Adair in an adjoining laboratory was able to supply Coombs with rabbit anti-human globulin sera. Sensitized red cells were agglutinated by the anti-sera whereas non-sensitized cells were not (33), and the Coombs' test was born. The Coombs' test is now carried out using specific monoclonal antibodies (Figure 4.5). Packman recounts that Carlo Moreschi had published a similar idea in 1908 but it had largely been ignored by the scientific community. Coombs acknowledged Moreschi in writing and during a lecture in Rome (34). The concept of antibodies reacting at body temperature (37°C) or strongly at 4°C was already accepted, and the clinical syndrome depended on the amount of antibody and its thermal amplitude.

Careful clinical evaluation also demonstrated that so-called autoimmune haemolytic anaemia (AIHA) was often associated with another disease. Over half of cases of AIHA arc associated with other diseases (35) and there can be an

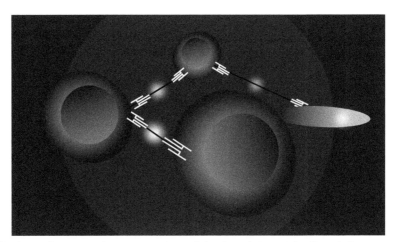

Fig. 4.5 A diagrammatic representations of the Coombs' test. The Coombs' reagent contains antibodies to Ig and/or complement and will form bridges so the cells can stick together.

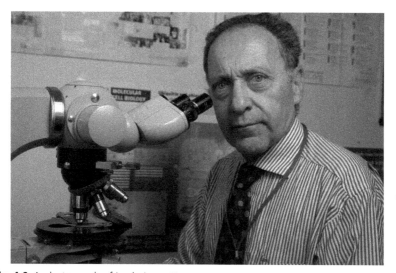

Fig. 4.6 A photograph of Lucio Luzzatto.

interval of many years after the AIHA is first diagnosed and the appearance of another disease (36). The most prominent haematologic disorders associated with AIHA appear to be chronic lymphocytic leukaemia and Hodgkin's lymphoma (36). Whether there is a generic predisposition to AIHA (only a minority of patients taking certain drugs develop AIHA) remains to be elucidated but there is a higher incidence of other autoimmune disorders in patients with AIHA than in patients without (37). Although corticosteroids and splenectomy have been advocated for many years for patients with AIHA, the therapeutic approach remains problematical in patients who fail to respond to either or both of these modalities. The use of the anti-CD20 drug rituximab has undoubtedly changed the outlook for many patients with AIHA (Figure 4.6). Chronic folic acid replacement is always recommended but patients with resistant disease still pose a problem for physicians.

Congenital spherocytes

Many physicians and even some haematologists refer to 'hereditary spherocytosis' (HS) as if it were a disease and not a syndrome. As we now know, there are many molecular lesions which can result in an abnormality of the red cell membrane, changing the erythrocyte from a bi-concave disc into a spherocyte. The clinical spectrum can vary from well-compensated haemolysis to life-threatening

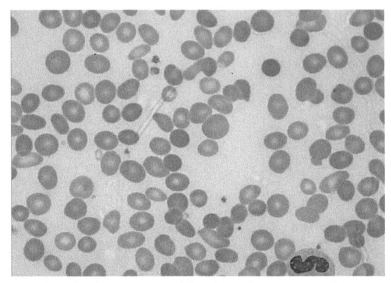

Fig. 4.7 A blood film from a patient with hereditary spherocytosis. In a two-dimensional view, spherocytes are seen as small dense red cells without the central pallor seen in normal red cells.

Reproduced from McCann S, Foà R, Smith O, and Conneally E., *Haematology: Clinical Cases Uncovered*, Second Edition, Wiley/Blackwell, Oxford, UK, Copyright © 2009, with permission from John Wiley and Sons Ltd.

neonatal haemolysis. Packman provides a beautiful example of an early description of the syndrome. (29). The paper by Constant Vanlair and J. R. Masius (38) provides a camera lucida drawing of spherocytes as visualized down a microscope, and Claude Wilson's cases from 1890 are probably the best examples of HS (39) (Figure 4.7).

The camera lucida

Many biologists used drawings of what they visualized down a microscope by using a camera lucida. This practice was maintained until the middle of the twentieth century but has since been replaced by digital photography. The principle of the camera lucida is the superimposition of the object being viewed on the surface upon which the artist/microscopist is drawing. This superimposition allows the artist/microscopist to duplicate any points on the object he/she wishes on the drawing surface, thus avoiding difficulties of perspective.

A lot has been written about the metabolic abnormalities in erythrocytes from patients with HS. The inability of red cells from patients with HS to withstand osmotic shock has been the basis for the osmotic fragility test (Figure 4.8).

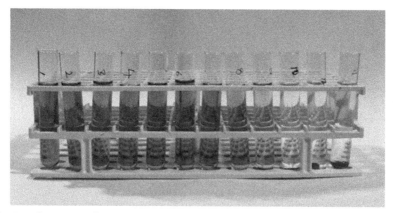

Fig. 4.8 The osmotic fragility test.

The osmotic fragility test measures the ability of red cells to resist osmotic shock (resistance to rupture when they are incubated in saline solutions). As normal red cells are bi-concave discs, they are more resistant to rupture than spherocytes are, as normal red cells have a larger surface area to volume ratio, compared to spherocytes. This resistance is reflected in the amount of haemoglobin released when red cells are incubated in 12 different solutions of saline, thus revealing any difference between the sensitivity of normal red cells and that of those from the patient's sample. Tube 12 contains normal saline, so no haemolysis is expected. As the number go down to 1, the saline becomes hypotonic and there is a gradual increase in cell rupture and release of haemoglobin. The result is expressed graphically in Figure 4.9.

The Coombs' test made it possible to distinguish congenital from acquired spherocytes. However, it was the description of the red cell cytoskeleton by Vincent Marchesi and colleagues (40, 41) which opened the door to the understanding of this syndrome and related red cell disorders.

Among the reasons the physiology of the erythrocyte is so well understood are the ready availability of blood samples and the relative ease of making red cell 'ghosts' which can then be studied. Erythrocytes are highly deformable and have the ability to return to their original shape. The plasma membrane is responsible for all of the cell's antigenic, transport, and mechanical characteristics (42), and splenic sequestration of abnormal red cells with reduced deformability accounts for the shortened lifespan and increased haemolysis in many red cell disorders. The nature of the plasma membrane and red cell deformability began to be understood following the report that micropipette aspiration could be used to measure erythrocyte 'stiffness' (43). Human red cells

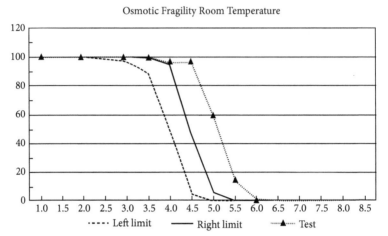

Fig. 4.9 The results of the osmotic fragility test.

undergo marked shape changes because of the structural organization of the plasma membrane. The red cell is remarkably elastic but is very sensitive to loss of plasma membrane, that is, a change in surface area (42). The red cell plasma membrane comprises an envelope composed of cholesterol and phospholipids; this envelope is anchored to a two-dimensional elastic network of skeletal proteins via tethering sites on cytoplasmic domains of transmembrane proteins embedded in the lipid bilayer. The major phospholipids are asymmetrically distributed, with phosphatidylcholine and sphingomyelin being mostly in the outer monolayer, and phosphatidylserine and phosphatidylethanolamine predominantly in the inner monolayer. The location of phosphatidylserine in the inner monolayer is necessary to protect erythrocytes from phagocytosis and facilitates passage through the microvasculature by inhibiting adhesion to vascular endothelium (42).

Membrane proteins function as transport proteins, adhesion proteins, signalling receptors, and blood group antigens. Band 3 (so-called because of its position on sodium dodecyl sulphate polyacrylamide gel electrophoresis) acts as the major anion and CO_2 transporter. The major red cell proteins are alpha spectrin, beta spectrin, actin, and Protein 4.1 R. Spectrin tetramer, the major structural component of the cytoskeleton, is formed by the lateral interaction of spectrin dimers. Protein 4.1 R facilitates the interaction between spectrin and actin. This cytoskeleton plays a critical role in preventing deformation-induced membrane fragmentation, which could occur when red cells experience high fluid shear stresses in the circulation.

In HS, hereditary eliptocytosis, hereditary ovalocytosis, and hereditary stomatocytosis, there are mutations in the membrane or skeletal proteins. HS can be inherited dominantly or nondominantly and, although it affects all ethnic groups, it is more common in northern Europeans than in other ethnic groups. Affected patients have splenomegaly, reticulocytosis, jaundice, and gall stones. The severity is very variable and it is not uncommon to see patients with well-compensated haemolysis and a normal haemoglobin level. Anaemia can be severe and can be exacerbated by folate deficiency secondary to chronic haemolysis or by parvovirus infection. All patients with HS have erythrocytes that have less surface area and are less deformable than normal erythrocytes and thus are trapped in the spleen and removed from the circulation. The loss of membrane is due to a defect in the gene encoding a protein which is involved in vertical linkages between the skeletal network and the membrane.

Interestingly, both hereditary eliptocytosis and hereditary ovalocytosis occur in areas where malaria is endemic. The prevalence of hereditary eliptocytosis approaches 2% in West Africa, and ovalocytosis has a prevalence of 5%-25% in South East Asia (44). Jarlim and colleagues reported two linked mutations in band 3 (45), and Che and colleagues deduced that the reduced rotational mobility of

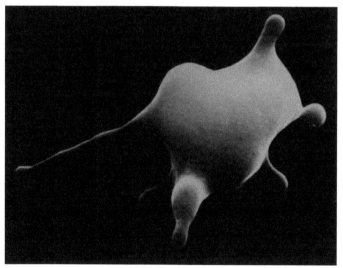

Fig. 4.10 A scanning electron microscopic photograph of acanthocytes, which are erythrocytes with elongated surface membrane projections.

band 3 in ovalocytes is a consequence of the formation of micro-aggregates, which are very probably induced by the mutation in the membrane-bound domain of ovalocytic band 3 (46). Didier Dhermy and colleagues (47) suggest that certain specific spectrin alleles might confer resistance to malaria.

Acanthocytes

Another acquired membrane abnormality is acanthocytosis. Cholesterol in the red cell membrane is in dynamic equilibrium with cholesterol in the plasma. In severe liver disease, there is a deficiency of the enzyme lecithin-cholesterol acetyltransferase (LCAT). Acanthocytosis may also be a familial disease due to mutations in the LCAT gene. The result of LCAT deficiency is an accumulation of cholesterol in the red cell membrane, with an increase in surface area leading to the formation of acanthocytes (Figure 4.10). These erythrocytes experience phagocytosis of their excess membrane in the spleen, and haemolysis ensues. Because of their increased surface area, the red cells have a decreased osmotic fragility, in contrast to the case for spherocytes.

Conclusion

Although the dangers of premature red cell destruction were recognized in ancient Greece, it took careful elucidation of erythrocyte physiology before the mechanisms underlying such destruction became clear. Conditions which lead to a shortened red cell lifespan may be very common (e.g. G6PD deficiency) or very rare (e.g. paroxysmal nocturnal haemoglobinuria). Whether anaemia ensues, the underlying intracellular, membrane, or immune modulation can be studied extensively because of easy access to blood samples. Careful clinical observations over time, together with painstaking laboratory investigations, have led to the understanding of these conditions, and this understanding has been of great benefit to geneticists, immunologists, haematologists, and most importantly to patients. Understanding of the underlying pathophysiology has allowed novel treatments to be developed which can be life-saving or significantly improve patients' quality of life.

References

1 Wintrobe MM. Blood, Pure and Eloquent. McGraw-Hill, New York, NY 1980.

2 Hajdu SI. A note from history: The discovery of blood cells. Annals of Clinical and Laboratory Science **33** (2): 237–8. 2003.

3 Donné A. De L'origine des globules du sang de leur mode de formation et leur fin. Comptes rendus hebdomadaires des séances de l'Académie des Sciences **14**: 366–8. 1842.

4   Degos L. Personal communication. 2014.

5   Dacie J. The Haemolytic Anaemias. **Volume I**. Churchill Livingstone, London, 1985.

6   Dressler LA. Ein Fall von intermittirender Albuminurie und Chromaturie. Archiv für pathologische Anatomie und Physiologie und für klinische Medicin **6** (2): 264–6. 1854.

7   Ashby W. The determination of the length of life of transfused red corpuscles in man. Journal of Experimental Medicine **29** (3): 267–81. 1919.

8   Beutler E. Glucose-6-phosphate dehydrogenase deficiency: A historical perspective. Blood **111** (1): 53–61. 2008.

9   Beutler E, Dern RJ, Alvin AS. The haemolytic effect of primaquine. VI. An in vitro test for erythrocytes to primaquine. Journal of Laboratory and Clinical Medicine **45** (1): 40–50. 1955.

10 Beutler E, Dern RJ, Flanagan CL, Alving AS. The haemolytic effect of primaquine. VII. Biochemical studies of drug-sensitive erythrocytes. Journal of Laboratory and Clinical Medicine **45** (2): 286–95. 1955.

11 Luzzatto L, Usanga EA, Reddy S. Glucose 6-phosphate deficient red cells: Resistance to malaria parasites. Science **164** (3881): 839–42. 1969.

12 Luzzatto L and Seneca E. G6PD deficiency: A classic example of pharmacogenetics with on-going clinical implications. British Journal of Haematology **164** (4): 469–80. 2014.

13 Parker CJ. Paroxysmal nocturnal hemoglobinuria: An historical overview. ASH Education Program Book **2008** (1): 93–103. 2008.

14 Crosby WH. Paroxysmal nocturnal hemoglobinuria: A classic description by Paul Strübing in 1882 and a bibliography of the disease. Blood **6** (3): 270–84. 1951.

15 Ham TH, Dingle JH. Studies on the destruction of red blood cells. II. Chronic hemolytic anemia with paroxysmal nocturnal hemoglobinuria: Certain immunological aspects of the haemolytic mechanism with special reference to serum complement. Journal of Clinical Investigation **18** (6): 657–72. 1939.

16 Hinz CF Jr, Jordan WS Jr, Pillemer L. The properdin system and immunity. IV. The hemolysis of erythrocytes from patients with paroxysmal nocturnal hemoglobinuria. Journal of Clinical Investigation **35** (5): 453–7. 1956.

17 Crosby WH. Paroxysmal nocturnal hemoglobinuria. Blood **8** (9): 769–812. 1953.

18 Rosse WF, Dacie JV. Immune lysis of normal human and paroxysmal nocturnal hemoglobinuria (PNH) red blood cells. I. The sensitivity of PNH red cells to lysis by complement and specific antibody. Journal of Clinical Investigation **45** (5): 736–48. 1966.

19 Rosse WF, Dacie JV. Immune lysis of normal human and paroxysmal nocturnal hemoglobimuria (PNH) red blood cells. II. The role of complement components in the increased sensitivity of PNH red cells to immune lysis. Journal of Clinical Investigation **45** (5): 749–57. 1966.

20 Hartman RC, Jenkins DE. The 'sugar-water test' for paroxysmal nocturnal hemoglobinuria. New England Journal of Medicine **275** (3): 155–7. 1966.

21 Luzzatto L, Nafa K. Genetics of PNH, in NS Young, J Moss, eds, Paroxysmal Nocturnal Hemoglobinuria and the Glycosylphosphatidylinositol-Linked Proteins. Academic Press, San Diego, CA, 2000, pp. 21–47.

22 Endo M, Ware RE, Vreeke TM, Singh SP, Howard TA, Tomita A, et al. Molecular basis of the heterogeneity of expression of glycosyl phosphatidylinositol anchored proteins in paroxysmal nocturnal hemoglobinuria. Blood **87** (6): 2456–557. 1996.

23 Hillmen P. The role of complement inhibition in PNH. ASH Education Program Book **2008** (1): 116–23. 2008.

24 Hillmen P, Young NS, Schubert J, Brodsky RA, Socié G, Muus P, et al. The complement inhibitor eculizumab in paroxysmal nocturnal hemoglobinuria. New England Journal of Medicine **355** (12): 1233–43. 2006.

25 Hillmen P, Muus P, Dührsen U, Risitano AM, Schubert J, Luzzatto L, et al. Effect of the complement inhibitor eculizumab on thromboembolism in patients with paroxysmal nocturnal hemoglobinuria. Blood **110** (12): 4123–8. 2007.

26 Rother RP, Bell L, Hillmen P, Gladwin MT. The clinical sequelae of intravascular hemolysis and extracellular plasma hemoglobin. A novel mechanism of human disease. Journal of the American Medical Association **293** (13): 1653–62. 2005.

27 LoBuglio AF, Cotran RS, Jandl JH. Red cells coated with immunoglobulin G: Binding and sphering by mononuclear cells in man. Science **158** (3808): 1582–5. 1967.

28 Huber H, Polley MJ, Lindscott WD, Fudenberg HH, Müller-Eberhard HJ. Human monocytes: Distinct receptor sites for the third component of complement and for immunoglobulin G. Science **162** (3859): 1281–3. 1968.

29 Packman CH. The spherocytic haemolytic anaemias. British Journal of Haematology **112** (4): 888–99. 2001.

30 Dreyfus C. Chronic hemolytic jaundice. A historical study. Bulletin of the New England Medical Center **4**: 122–8. 1942.

31 Dacie JV. The immune haemolytis anaemias: A century of exciting progress in understanding. British Journal of Haematology **114** (4): 770–85. 2001.

32 Coombs RRA. Historical note: Past present and future of the antiglobulin test. Vox Sanguinis **74** (2): 67–73. 1998.

33 Coombs RRA, Mourant AE, Race RR. A new test for the detection of weak and 'incomplete' Rh agglutinins. British Journal of Experimental Pathology **26** (4): 255–66. 1945.

34 Petz LD, Garratty G. Acquired Immune Hemolytic Anemias. Churdhill Livingstone, New York, 1980.

35 Conley CL. Immunologic precursors of autoimmune hematologic disorders. Autoimmune hematologic disorders. Autoimmune hemolytic anemia and thrombocytopenic purpura. Johns Hopkins Medical Journal **149** (3): 101–9. 1981.

36 Pirovsky B. Autoimmunization and the Autoimmune Hemolytic Anaemias. Williams & Wilkins, Baltimore, MD, 1969.

37 Luzzatto L. Personal communication 2014.

38 Vanlair C, Masius JR. De la microcythémie. Bulletin de l'Academie Royal de Médicin Belgique **5**: 515–613 1871.

39 Wilson C. Some cases showing hereditary enlargement of the spleen. Transactions of the Clinical Society of London **26**: 163–71. 1890.

40 Marchesi VT, Steers E Jr. Selective solubilization of a protein component of the red cell membrane. Science **159** (3811): 203–4. 1968.

41 Steck TL, Fairbanks G, Wallach DF. Disposition of the major proteins in the isolated erythrocyte membrane. Proteolytic dissection. Biochemistry **10** (13): 2617–24. 1971.

42 Mohandas N, Gallagher PG. Red cell membrane: Past, present and future. Blood **112** (10): 3939–48. 2008.

43 **Rand RP, Burton AC**. Mechanical properties of the red cell membrane: I. Membrane stiffness and intracellular pressure. Biophysics Journal **4** (2): 115–35. 1964.

44 **Amato D, Booth PB**. Hereditary ovalocytosis in Melanesians. Papua and New Guinea Medical Journal **20** (1): 26–32. 1977.

45 **Jarlim P, Palek J, Amato D, Hassan K, Sapak P, Nurse GT, et al**. Deletion in erythrocyte band 3 gene in malaria-resistant Southeast Asian ovalocytosis. Proceedings of the National Academy of Sciences of the United States of America **88** (24): 11022–6. 1991.

46 **Che A, Cherry RJ, Bannister LH, Dluzewski, AR**. Aggregation of band 3 in hereditary ovalocytic red blood cell membranes. Electron microscopy and protein rotational diffusion studies. Journal of Cell Science **105** (3): 655–60. 1993.

47 **Dhermy D, Schrével J, Lecomte MC**. Spectrin-based skeleton in red blood cells and malaria. Current Opinion in Hematology **14** (3): 198–202. 2007.

Chapter 5

Blood and the hidden virus

Of men, monkeys, and lepidopterists: The development of anti-D

A major achievement in the history of blood transfusion was discovery of the Rh blood groups. The foundation for this discovery way laid in 1939, when Philip Levine (1900–87) (who worked with Karl Landsteiner) and Rufus Stetson described the now-famous case of a woman who experienced a transfusion reaction when she was transfused with blood from her husband, even though they both had Group O blood (1). Levine and Stetson subsequently discovered an antibody in the woman's blood which reacted against her husband's red cells. When they then found that the woman had just been delivered of a stillborn baby with severe haemolytic disease, Levine and Stetson suggested that the husband and wife had another antigen on their red cells, apart from the O antigen, and that thus the blood group of the fetus was slightly different from that of the mother. They then hypothesized that, when some red cells from the fetus had crossed the placenta into the mother's circulation during fetal development, her immune system had recognized these red cells as being different and made antibodies against them and that these antibodies had then crossed the placenta in the opposite direction and destroyed the red cells in the fetus, causing it to be stillborn. This work paved the way for our full understanding of the Rh blood groups and Rh-positive babies who suffer from erythroblastosis fetalis, more accurately called haemolytic disease of the newborn (HDNB).

HDNB and the Rh factor

In the early seventeenth century, a French midwife, Louise Bourgeois, delivered twins, of whom one was hydropic (a sign of prenatal heart failure due to severe anaemia; indicated by gross swelling and often accompanied by premature death), and the other died after a few hours, with rapidly developing jaundice. This case was undoubtedly the first description of HDNB (2). In the early twentieth century, George Auden, Harvey Hubbard, and Henning von Gierke described diseases which were certainly HDNB (3). In 1932 Louis Diamond and colleagues recognized that hydrops foetalis, severe neonatal jaundice, and delayed anaemia of the newborn shared a pathological process (4). However, it was not until 1938 that Ruth Darrow, a New York pathologist, hypothesized the immunological nature of HDNB (5).

It has been claimed that, in the case of HDNB, 'in the span of little more than 20 years, the aetiology of a mysterious and unknown disease is discovered, its immunological pathogenesis determined, [and] an efficient therapy . . . is introduced' (6). Around the same time that Darrow proposed her hypothesis, Landsteiner and his colleagues injected blood from rhesus monkeys into rabbits, and the rabbits produced an antibody. This antibody reacted with red cells from approximately 85% of the individuals examined; such individuals were termed 'Rh positive'. Individuals with red cells that did not react with the antibody, around 15% of those examined, were termed 'Rh negative' (7, 8). It was subsequently found that the presence of a difference between the Rh blood groups of the mother and the fetus accounts for the majority of cases of HDNB (9). Levine then noticed that, if there were major blood group differences between the mother and the father of the affected infant, the severity of HDNB appeared to be reduced (10). He reasoned that, in those cases, the red cells which 'leaked' from the fetus into the mother's circulation were so different that they were immediately destroyed before the mother could make antibodies to the Rh blood group. His observations were confirmed by Robert Race and Ruth Sanger (11) and by the experiments of Kurt Stern and colleagues (12). Levine, who had migrated to the United States from Minsk, Belarus (at that time part of the former Soviet Union), at the age of 8 years, later shared the prestigious Lasker Award with Landsteiner and Alexander Wiener in 1946 for his work on the Rh factor.

Butterflies and babies

There are many names associated with HDNB but Sir Cyril Clarke is probably the name that most people associate with the following remarkable story. As a child, he was an enthusiastic lepidopterist, and he rekindled his interest in the subject during World War II, when he spent a year in a naval hospital in Australia. His interest in butterflies also led to a life-long interest in genetics. (13). In Liverpool he enjoyed a life-long collaboration with Phillip M. Sheppard, who became Professor of Genetics while Clarke became Professor of Medicine. They went on to dispel the myth surrounding blood groups and peptic ulcer disease (14, 15) but it was the similarities between the inheritance of Rh blood groups and that of mimetic patterns in butterflies that stimulated their interest in Rh blood groups: in both cases, the genes encoding phenotypes are located on the same chromosome and are tightly linked, with occasional crossover producing rare genotypes.

In 1959, Alvin Zipursky and colleagues showed that, by using the Kleihauer technique, they were able to detect fetal cells in the maternal circulation and thus quantify the risk of immunization (16, 17). The following year, Ronald

Finn, at that time working on his MD thesis with Clarke, suggested that these fetal cells might be destroyed in the maternal circulation by a suitable antibody (18). In the same year Vincent J. Freda (19), an obstetrician in the United States, proposed that, if a woman were given anti-Rh antibodies, she could be prevented from making her own antibodies against the Rh factor of the fetus; in other words, the injected antibody would 'block' the mother from manufacturing anti-Rh antibodies. Freda was familiar with experiments that had been carried out in 1900 by a microbiologist called Theobald Smith and which demonstrated the blocking of antibodies in rabbits (20). Clarke came to a similar conclusion because he knew that in butterfly breeding a 'blocking factor' could prevent the expression of wing colour inheritance (13).

Clarke went on to inject Rh-positive cells, together with anti-Rh antibodies, into Rh-negative male volunteers; such an experiment certainly would not be carried out nowadays. Nonetheless, in 1961 they reported the successful blocking of anti-Rh antibodies in the volunteers (21). Interestingly, in a review of his work (13), Clarke recounts a report by John Jewkes and colleagues that Eugene Hamilton, a doctor from St. Louis, revealed in 1967 that, having read the 1961 article by Clarke et al., from 1962 onwards he had been immunizing mothers using plasma prepared from sensitized mothers with no history of jaundice and that the immunization had proven effective in preventing HDNB (22).

These experiments and the work of many others resulted in the manufacture of anti-Rh antibodies—specifically, antibodies against the D antigen of the Rh blood group system—in a very small volume, which was then injected intramuscularly into Rh-negative mothers shortly after delivering Rh-positive babies. There were many discussions and position papers about the correct dose of anti-D, the correct type of antibody to use, and the method of administration. Moreover, in 1967 Nevin Hughes-Jones provided a method which gave more accurate information about the efficiency of anti-D than simply measuring the titre of the antibody did (23). Thus, the world was transformed for parents and babies with Rh factor complications. Clarke made a very interesting point at the end of his 1989 review (13), saying: 'The Liverpool work is a good example of research starting out as "useless"... but in fact paying off later. It could never have been planned . . . Treasure your contradictions'.

Alas, like many scientific breakthroughs, things did not run as smoothly as might be hoped.

The tragedy of hepatitis and anti-D

In 1994 a discovery was made which was to cause great human suffering, stress, and loss of trust and result in a critical fall in donor numbers in Ireland.

Tragically, it was found that in two countries, Germany and Ireland the anti-D blood product used to prevent Rh-associated HDNB had become contaminated during the 1970s with the then unidentified hepatitis C virus. This contamination was in part caused by production technology that used an ethanol step which differed significantly from that in the classical Cohn process of plasma fractionation and in part due to poor selection of donors (24). In the case of Ireland, anti-D was prepared at that time by the Blood Transfusion Service Board (BTSB). Anti-D was made from the plasma of male Rh-negative volunteers who had been immunized with Rh-positive red cells, plasma from women who had been immunized through pregnancy, or plasma from individuals immunized through blood transfusion, as the plasma of this latter group contained large amounts of anti-D. Because of its different production method, this anti-D immunoglobulin could be given intravenously rather than intramuscularly. In addition, the anti-D produced in this way was very effective in preventing women from becoming immunized.

Unfortunately, the women who had been immunized against Rh during pregnancy had been treated with 'plasma exchange', where their plasma had been removed and then replaced by normal plasma in the hope that their babies would be born unaffected. In 1976 one of these women became jaundiced; at that time, it was believed she was infected with what was thought to be hepatitis A. As hepatitis A was not thought at that time to be transmitted by blood products, when she appeared to have recovered, her plasma was again used in the production of anti-D. Unfortunately, it turned out that one of the units of plasma she had received during her plasma exchange treatment when she was pregnant had been contaminated with hepatitis C (unidentified at that time). A number of women who received anti-D made from her plasma became jaundiced. They and the original patient were then investigated for the only other hepatitis virus known at the time, hepatitis B, which was very serious and sometimes fatal, but none of the women showed signs of hepatitis B infection. Therefore, the manufacture of anti-D recommenced; subsequently, many young women who received the anti-D became infected with hepatitis C. Some of these also became blood donors and thereby inadvertently introduced hepatitis C into the blood supply.

Hepatitis C isolated

In 1989 the hepatitis C virus was finally isolated in California. Its discovery was hailed across the world. At that time, many doctors and scientists believed that the hepatitis C virus would turn out to be the missing link in diseases such as aplastic anaemia (although it later transpired that this was not the case) and would explain the abnormal liver blood tests seen in many patients with haemophilia. It turned out that hepatitis C produced infections which remained asymptomatic for years. At that time, there was no test for the virus itself, so the presence of antibodies in a person's blood was taken as evidence of infection. The original blood samples from the jaundiced women in Ireland from the 1970s were then tested for hepatitis C antibodies and found to be positive. The medical director of the BTSB in Dublin was informed but, unfortunately, no action was taken.

Blood banks worldwide began to test donors to try to find out how common hepatitis C infection was in the general population and to prevent its transmission by blood transfusion. The BTSB introduced hepatitis C testing in October 1991, around the same time as it was introduced in Britain, in order to determine the prevalence of hepatitis in the community. Although blood donors were generally relatively young and deemed to be otherwise healthy, a unit of the BTSB discovered a rather high and unexpected number of donors with antibodies to hepatitis C. On close inspection in late 1993 and early 1994, it became clear that the majority of these donors were Rh-negative women. Alarm bells were sounded, because the one thing these women had in common was that they had been treated with anti-D in the past. The medical director in Dublin was informed and the results of the original tests on the women who had become jaundiced after treatment with anti-D became available. Anti-D manufactured by the Irish Blood Transfusion Board was recalled and a new, safe product, was imported from Canada. Over the weekend of 18 February 1994, a nationwide screening programme to offer testing to all recipients of anti-D was launched, with huge media coverage. Unfortunately, many women were found to have signs of chronic hepatitis C infection. The national medical director of the BTSB resigned. There was a hue and cry in the media. The BTSB then began a series of retrospective transfusion investigations to try to identify the source of the hepatitis infection. The staff worked extremely hard under very difficult circumstances but the public began to lose faith in the BTSB, and the blood supply was threatened.

Blood supply threatened

It was a very difficult time for all involved. Everybody worked hard to maintain the morale in the BTSB and to reassure the public that blood from donors was being tested adequately for hepatitis C infection. The media had a field day and there was a lot of misinformation published. Journalists wrote articles about hepatitis C almost daily. A prominent politician suggested that the BTSB should be closed and all staff dismissed. It was pointed out that there would be no blood supply in Ireland for months or years if this line of action was followed. The service did not close but tried to make sure that all testing and other protocols were up to date. The state of the blood supply was precarious, as all the adverse publicity made collection of adequate amounts of blood difficult. Hospitals continued to use blood products for surgery and for patients receiving chemotherapy. All the royal colleges, including the Royal College of Physicians, the Royal College of Surgeons, and the Institute of Obstetrics and Gynaecology in Ireland, refused to make a statement saying that blood was now safe, even though they continued to oversee its use. The Irish government set up inquiries (24, 25), appointed a large number of hepatologists, and provided compensation, via a tribunal, for people who had become infected through blood transfusion, but the damage done continued for some time afterwards. It is estimated that 1055 women were infected via anti-D, and 412 people by blood transfusion. Five recipients of infected anti-D (0.6%) have developed liver cancer, and 13 (1.6%) have died from liver disease (26). Thankfully, the incidence of serious complications in Germany and Ireland was low, probably because the recipients were young healthy females. In recent years, chronically infected patients have responded well to new antiviral drug combinations.

In Germany, although it was reported that a number of individuals received jail sentences, there was no public enquiry or state financial support for victims.

Mad cows and blood

At the same time that the blood supply was being threatened by hepatitis C contamination, a new threat was emerging. The decision to feed cattle, which are herbivores, with bonemeal turned out to be a very expensive mistake and produced widespread fear of a human epidemic of 'mad cow disease'. The bonemeal used was manufactured from carcasses and the cooked and ground leftovers of the slaughter of cattle and sheep. It was then was used in cattle feed instead of soybean-derived protein, as it was cheaper than the plant-based protein, and protein, together with hormones and antibiotics, was given because it increased animal weight and therefore the sale value. The first animal with mad cow disease died in the United Kingdom in 1986 and, the following year, it became clear that bovine spongiform encephalopathy was the cause of mad cow disease. The disease was found predominantly in the United Kingdom, although there were substantial numbers of infected cattle in Ireland, France, Spain, and Portugal (27).

Could mad cow disease be transmitted by blood or blood products?

Variant Creutzfeldt–Jakob disease (vCJD) is the human equivalent of BSE. It is one of a small number of invariably fatal neurological diseases (spongiform encephalopathies) associated with an abnormal form of prion protein (Figure 5.1).

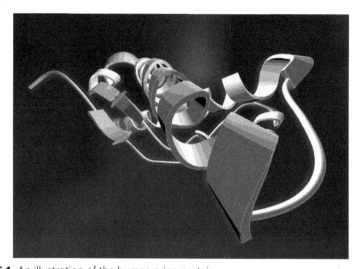

Fig. 5.1 An illustration of the human prion protein.

Reproduced with permission from Wellcome Library, London. Image ID: B0009547. Credit: Anna Tanczos/Wellcome Images. Copyright © 2014 Anna Tanczos.

It is now believed that vCJD spread to humans via cattle infected with BSE (28). The question for haematologists and those involved in public health was: will blood or blood product transfusion spread this disease and will there be many deaths? Initially, it seemed like it would be another Armageddon, as with HIV and hepatitis C; but subsequent events and actions have perhaps changed the outcome for the better.

Universal leucodepletion

The evidence strongly suggests that removal of white cells, a process termed leucodepletion, at the time of collection of donated blood reduces the risk of transmission of vCJD via the transfusion of blood or blood products. Leukodepletion was introduced in the United Kingdom and Ireland in 1999, and plasma derivatives have been either fractionated from imported plasma or manufactured using recombinant technology. Fresh frozen plasma is now imported, and recipients of blood components have been excluded from donating blood in the United Kingdom since 2004. The total number of people who contracted vCJD via blood transfusion in the United Kingdom is 3, and all of them are deceased, whereas the total number of cases of vCJD thought to be caused by eating contaminated beef products is 174 (29). There have been no cases of blood-borne transmission of vCJD outside the United Kingdom.

Is there a screening test for vCJD?

Unlike other infectious diseases transmitted by blood or blood products, there is *no* screening test for vCJD. There are a number of reasons for this fact. The first reason is that the pathobiology of vCJD is peculiar. The prion protein (PrP) is a naturally occurring membrane glycoprotein and is the product of a gene present in all vertebrates. The abnormal form of the protein, termed PrP^{Sc}, causes the destruction of brain cells. It is infectious, and the beta form is resistant to degradation. Within the PrP gene, Codon 129, which can code for methionine or valine, has a major effect on the susceptibility to prion disease. About 40% of the population in the United Kingdom is homozygous for methionine at position 129; however, to date, all victims of vCJD have had this genotype; thus, having this genotype may shorten the incubation period of the infection (29). The origin of BSE is still disputed, and theories vary from a chance mutation in an animal sent for slaughter and used for the manufacture of bonemeal, to the use of insecticides, to autoimmunity (29).

The second reason why there is no screening test for vCJD available to blood transfusion centres at present is that, since vCJD does not provoke an immune response (i.e. antibody formation), the time-honoured method of detecting infection via antibody titre cannot be employed. The third reason is that, since the disease is thought to arise from protein misfolding rather than from a genetic mutation, nucleic acid testing is not possible. Edgeworth and colleagues (30) have recently provided a prototype blood test for vCJD in symptomatic individuals but as yet we do not have a test for asymptomatic prion infection. Even if we did have such a test, the incubation period could be as long as 30 years, and no treatment is currently available.

Finally, in an interesting editorial (31), William Murphy, the national medical director of the BTSB in 2012, pointed out that the health economics applied to the introduction of new drugs are different from those applied to the risk of transmitting infection via blood transfusions: if the modelling of health economics used to evaluate the cost-effectiveness of a new drug were applied to blood transfusion, testing for HIV, hepatitis B, hepatitis C, syphilis, and human T-lymphotropic virus type 1 and type 2 would be abandoned. However, such a decision would clearly not be acceptable as health policy. As he stated, 'Public perception . . . sets different values on public safety than on drug costs'. He also commented that luck had been far more important than skill in preventing a much larger vCJD disaster than actually occurred, because there was poor transmissibility of BSE to humans via the oral route.

Whatever one's views on blood transfusion and the relative risks of spreading disease, the practice of feeding meat to herbivores seems at the very least a strange thing to do and no doubt reflects human avarice to increase profits at all costs.

Some people don't want blood transfusions

Although the threat of infection via blood transfusion is real, there are many people who abjure being transfused with blood or blood products, regardless of their safety. The most well-known group which refuses blood transfusion is Jehovah's Witnesses. The name Jehovah's Witnesses evolved in 1931 from the Bible Student Movement of the late nineteenth century. There are 7.9 million followers engaged in evangelism, and 19.2 million attend the annual memorial services (32). The headquarters of the organization is in Brooklyn, New York. From the perspective of haematology, the most widely known attitude of Jehovah's Witnesses is to refuse to donate or receive blood transfusions. This stance is based on the belief that the Bible forbids the ingestion of human blood. The prohibition includes red cells, white cells, platelets, and plasma. Substances such as albumin, immunoglobulins, and factor concentrates are not absolutely forbidden and may be accepted at the discretion of the individual. In the case of children (minors) the courts usually overrule parents, and blood transfusion is given if indicated.

Bloodless surgery

Can you carry out serious surgery without the administration of blood or blood products? David Ott and Denton Cooley reviewed their experience in operating on Jehovah's Witnesses in 1977 (33), and a review appeared in 2005 by Manjit Gohel and colleagues (34). Gohel predicted at that time that 'bloodless surgery' would be the norm; however, this situation has not come about yet. True, blood transfusion has fallen by about 10% in the United States, following reports of a poorer outcome from elective surgery if patients received blood transfusion than if they did not. However, although immunological studies may show a suppressive effect of surgery-related transfusion, it should be pointed out that the poorer outcome associated with transfusion may be due to the fact that patients who require blood transfusion during surgery are already in a higher-risk group than those who do not (35). It also needs to be remembered that, by 2014, the majority of blood transfusions (>50%) in the Western world were for medical indications, trauma, or obstetrical indications (36).

It seems that a preoperative haemoglobin level of 70 g/l is sufficient to warrant 'bloodless surgery'. The 'holy grail' of autologous blood transfusion has also failed to fulfil its promise (37). At first glance, it seems the ideal solution; however, human error, the fact that many recipients of autologous transfusion also receive allogeneic blood, and the cost of procurement and storage all militate against its popular use. As Murphy said to me in 2014: 'Autologous blood transfusion—a huge fad in the 1990s—is more or less discontinued everywhere now. Some still goes on in the US, but everyone there is trying to get out of it' (37). The 2011 National Blood Collection and Utilization Survey Report by the US Department of Health and Human Services supports these views. The total number of blood collections in the United States decreased by 9% since 2008, and the number of red cells collected by apheresis increased by 2.7%. The number of autologous transfusions decreased by 55%. As a corollary, the number of red cell transfusions fell by 8% and, likewise, plasma transfusions decreased by 13.5%. These reductions were achieved via the implementation of a 'Patient Blood Management Program' and, in 2011, 30% of hospitals reported they had such a programme in place (38). A long-term worry might be that such a programme might cause doctors to become totally protocol driven and be unable to use their clinical judgement. However, during a recent discussion with Darrell Triulzi, Director of the Division of Transfusion Medicine at the University of Pittsburgh, he emphasized to me, that although there was a concerted effort to reduce unnecessary red cell transfusions, the doctor could always override the recommendations of the 'transfusion committee'.

References

1 **Levine P, Stetson RE**. An unusual case of intra-group agglutination. Journal of the American Medical Association **112** (2): 126–7. 1939.

2 **Bowman JM**. Hemolytic disease of the newborn. Vox Sanguinis **70** (Suppl 3): 620–67. 1996.

3 **Reali G**. Forty years of anti-D immunoprophylaxis. Blood Transfusion **5** (1): 3–6. 2007.

4 **Diamond LK, Blackfan KD, Baty JM**. Erythroblastosis fetalis and its association with universal edema of the fetus, icterus gravis neonatorum, and anemia of the newborn. Journal of Pediatrics **1** (3): 269–309. 1932.

5 **Darrow RR**. Icterus gravis (erythroblastosis) neonatorum: An examination of etiologic considerations. Archives of Pathology: **25**; 378–417. 1938.

6 **Velati C**. A survey of the current use of anti-D immunoprophylaxis and the incidence of haemolytic disease of the newborn in Italy. Blood Transfusion **5** (1) 7–14. 2007.

7 **Landsteiner K, Weiner AS**. An agglutinable factor in human blood recognized by immune sera for rhesus blood. Experimental Biology and Medicine (Maywood, NJ) **43** (1): 223–8. 1940.

8 **Landsteiner K, Weiner AS**. Studies on an agglutinogen (Rh) in human blood reacting with anti-rhesus sera and with human isoantibodies. Journal of Experimental Medicine **74** (4): 309–20. 1941.

9 **Levine P, Burnham L, Katzin EM, Vogel P**. The role of iso-immunization in the pathogenesis of erythroblastosis fetalis. American Journal of Obstetrics and Gynecology **42** (6): 925–37. 1941.

10 **Levine P**. Serological factors as possible causes in spontaneous abortions. Journal of Heredity **34** (3): 71–80. 1943.

11 **Race RR, Sanger R**. Blood Groups in Man. Blackwell, Oxford, 1950.

12 **Stern K, Goodman HS, Berger M**. Experimental isoimmunization to hemoantigens in man. Journal of Immunology **87** (2): 189–98. 1961.

13 **Clarke CA**. Preventing rhesus babies: The Liverpool research and follow up. Archives of Disease in Childhood **64** (12): 1734–40. 1989.

14 **Clarke CA, Edwards DW, Haddock DRW, Howel-Evans AW, McConnell RB, Sheppard PM**. ABO blood groups and secretor character in duodenal ulcer: Population and sibship studies. British Medical Journal **2**: 725–31. 1956.

15 **Clarke CA, Donohue WTA, McConnell RB, Martindale JH, Sheppard PM**. Blood groups and disease: Previous transfusions as a potential source of error in blood typing. British Medical Journal **1**: 1734–6. 1962.

16 **Zipursky A, Hull A, White FD, Israels LG**. Foetal erythrocytes in the maternal circulation. Lancet **273** (7070): 451–2. 1959.

17 **Kleihauer E, Braun H, Betke K**. Demonstration von fetalem Hämoglobin in den Erythrocyten eines Blutausstrichs. Klinische Wochenschrift **35** (12): 637–8. 1957.

18 **Finn R**. Erythroblastosis. Lancet **1** (9): 526. 1960.

19 **Freda VJ, Gorman JG, Pollack W**. Successful prevention of experimental Rh sensitization in man with anti-Rh gamma2-globulin antibody preparations. Transfusion **4** (1): 26–32. 1960.

20 **Smith T**. Variation among pathogenic bacteria. Journal of the Boston Society of Medical Sciences **4** (5): 95–105. 1900.

21 **Finn R, Clarke CA, Donohoe WTA, McConnell RB, Sheppard PM, Lehane D, et al**. Experimental studies on the prevention of Rh haemolytic disease. Br Med J **1**: 1486–90. 1961.

22 **Jewkes J, Sawers D, Stillerman R**. The Sources of Invention. Second edition. Macmillan, London, 1969.

23 **Hughes-Jones NC**. The estimation of the concentration and equilibrium constant of anti-D. Immunology **12** (5): 265–71. 1967.

24 **Finlay TA**. Report of the tribunal into the Blood Transfusion Service Board. Government Stationery Office, Dublin, 1997.

25 Communicable Disease Surveillance Centre. Tribunal report on outbreak of hepatitis C infection due to contaminated anti-D in Republic of Ireland sheds light on natural history of infection. Euro Surveill **1** (4): http://www.eurosurveillance.org/ViewArticle.aspx?ArticleId=1101. 1997.

26 Health Protection Surveillance Centre. National Hepatitis C Database for Infection Acquired through Blood and Blood Products. http://www.hpsc.ie/A-Z/Hepatitis/HepatitisC/HepatitisCDatabase/BaselineandFollow-upReports/, 2011.

27 **Bennett P, Daraktchiev W**. vCJD and Transfusion of Blood Components: An Updated Risk Assessment. Health Protection Analytical Team, Department of Health, London, 2013.

28 The University of Edinburgh. The National CJD Research and Surveillance Unit (NCJDRSU). http://www.cjd.ed.ac.uk/, 2012.

29 Lord Phillips of Worth Matravens. Lessons from the BSE inquiry. Journal of the Foundation for Science and Technology **17** (2): 3–4. 2001.

30 Edgemorth JA, Framer M, Sicilia A, Tavares P, Beck J, Campbell T, et al. Detection of prion infection in variant Creuzfeldt-Jakob disease: A blood-based assay. Lancet **377** (9764): 487–93. 2011.

31 Murphy W. Of mad cows and bolted horses: The economics of blood safety. Transfusion **52** (11): 2278–81. 2012.

32 Kosmin BA, Ariela Keysar, A. American Religious Identification Survey (ARIS 2008). Trinity College, Hartford, CT, 2008.

33 Ott DA, Cooley DA. Cardiovascular surgery in Jehovah's Witnesses: Report of 542 operations without blood transfusions. Journal of the American Medical Association **238** (12): 1256–8. 1977.

34 Gohel MS, Bulbulia RA, Slim FJ, Poskitt KR, Whyman MR. How to approach major surgery where patients refuse blood transfusion (including Jehovah's Witnesses). Annals of the Royal College of Surgeons of England **87** (1): 3–14. 2005.

35 Chinea R, Greenberg R, White I, Sacham-Shmueli E, Mahagna H, Avital S. Preoperative blood transfusion in cancer patients undergoing laparoscopic colorectal resection: Risk factors and impact on survival. Techniques in Coloproctology **17** (5): 549–54. 2013.

36 Etchason J, Petz L, Keeler E, Calhoun L, Kleinman S, Snider C, et al. The cost effectiveness of preoperative blood donations. New England Journal of Medicine **332** (11): 719–24. 1995.

37 Murphy W. Personal communication. 2014.

38 The United States Department of Health and Human Services. The 2011 National Blood Collection and Utilization Survey Report. http://www.hhs.gov/ash/bloodsafety/2011-nbcus.pdf, 2011.

Chapter 6

Radiation and transplantation
Towards an understanding of stem cells

The Manhattan Project

There is a paradoxical relationship between ionizing radiation and leukaemia. On the one hand, we know that exposure to high doses of ionizing radiation causes leukaemia; yet, the preparative regimens for stem cell transplantation, which can cure leukaemia, often specify total body irradiation. How did this relationship begin? The story of bone marrow transplantation or, as it is now called, stem cell transplantation, goes back to Los Alamos, New Mexico, and the 'Trinity' project.

It was early on a May morning in 1945 when the project leader J. Robert Oppenheimer (1904–67) and his colleagues set off to witness the first atomic explosion in history. Years had been spent preparing for this moment as they drove in the desert of New Mexico, from Los Alamos, to the 'Trinity' site, where the bomb, nicknamed 'The Gadget', would be detonated. The outcome remained uncertain. As the device exploded, they witnessed a most terrifying sight, of which Oppenheimer said years later, being reminded of an ancient Hindu text: 'I am become Death, the destroyer of worlds' (1).

Although the development of the atomic bomb was the result of a war initiative, the discovery was to have major biological significance. The story started some years before World War II. In the early 1930s, Ernest T. S. Walton (1903–95), a graduate of Trinity College, Dublin, and John Cockcroft (1897–1967), a graduate of Manchester University, while working at the Cavendish Laboratory in Cambridge, built an apparatus that split the nuclei of lithium atoms by bombarding them with a stream of protons accelerated inside a high-voltage tube. The splitting of the lithium nuclei produced helium nuclei and so began a scientific race that led ultimately to the first atomic bomb and the Nobel Prize for Physics for Walton and Cockcroft in 1951. In 2014, a beautiful sculpture commemorating Ernest Walton's work, created by the Irish artist Eilís O'Connell, was unveiled in Trinity College, Dublin (Figure 6.1).

However when two German physicists, Otto Hahn (1879–1968) and Fritz Strassmann (1902–80), published experimental results about bombarding uranium with neutrons in December 1938, the US government established a secret

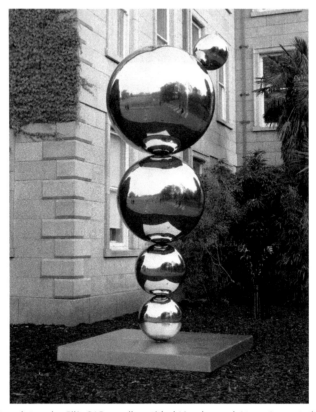

Fig. 6.1 A sculpture by Eilís O'Connell, entitled 'Apples and Atoms'; created in 2013, to celebrate the accomplishments of the Nobel Laureate Ernest T. S. Walton. The sculpture is made of mirror-polished stainless steel and is 420 cm high; it currently resides in the Trinity College Dublin Art Collections.

laboratory with the most brilliant scientists available, to develop an atomic bomb to counteract the nuclear threat from Germany. The American fear was probably well founded, as the eminent physicist Albert Einstein wrote several letters to President Franklin D. Roosevelt, urging him to establish a nuclear capability ahead of the Germans (2). Interestingly, the atomic bomb and the biological significance of ionizing radiation became intrinsically linked as the story of stem cells in bone marrow began to unfold: these two apparently unconnected events became interdependent.

One of the many ironies of the attempt by Adolf Hitler and Benito Mussolini to develop a 'master race' and the perfect state in Europe was to drive many of the best scientists in Germany and Italy to America. This allowed the US government to gather the largest group of scientists ever assembled up to that time in a single location, with the specific mission of developing an atomic bomb. The remote site chosen was Los Alamos in New Mexico and the project was named the 'Manhattan Project', after the Manhattan District of War Department. The unusual sequestration of scientists and their spouses in very restricted conditions with a foreboding atmosphere was under the direction of Leslie Groves (1898–1970) (2). Groves was a capable administrator, who oversaw the Manhattan Project following his supervision of the construction of the Pentagon. Groves retired from the army in 1948 and was promoted to Lieutenant General, backdated to 1945. Oak Ridge in Tennessee was the site for the enrichment of uranium. At its peak, the Manhattan Project employed 130,000 people in three countries (the United States, Canada, and the United Kingdom) and cost almost $22 billion in current value.

Two of the best remembered names from the Manhattan Project are Oppenheimer and Enrico Fermi (1901–54). Oppenheimer was an American theoretical physicist, Professor of Physics at the University of California in Berkeley, and scientific director of the Manhattan Project. Fermi, an Italian physicist, left Rome for America in 1939 shortly after receiving the Nobel Prize as one of the world's greatest experts in nuclear physics. Fermi was educated in Pisa. He also worked in Göttingen and Leiden before his appointment at the University of Rome as Professor of Theoretical Physics. He was recognised as the world's greatest expert on neutrons and his work led to the first nuclear controlled reaction. Oppenheimer's family had come to America in 1869 and lived in a very upmarket apartment on West 94th street when Robert was born. The family was well off and employed a governess, a chauffeur, and three live-in maids (1). According to Oppenheimer's biographer Ray Monk, the Oppenheimers, like many German-Americans, tried to lose all traces of their accents and ethnicity during World War I.

Oppenheimer, following a stellar undergraduate career in Harvard, went to Cambridge, UK, and then to the University of Göttingen in Germany. He subsequently returned to the United States and divided his time between Harvard and the California Institute of Technology (also known as Caltech). Like many people in the 1930s, he developed tuberculosis and spent some time recovering in a ranch in New Mexico. During this time, he developed a love of the New Mexican desert, which he retained for the remainder of his life. In spite of his enormous contribution to physics, Oppenheimer had a rather tragic life and, like many others in the United States, fell foul of the backlash against those who held liberal left-wing views during and after World War II. Although he was nominated for the Nobel Prize, it was never awarded and this fact may reflect the effect of his political leanings on his career. As with many extremely gifted individuals, opinions about him varied; descriptions of him ranged from 'aloof' to 'pretentious' and 'insecure'. In spite of being the scientific director of the Manhattan Project, Oppenheimer was the subject of constant surveillance by the FBI because he had reportedly organized a number of fund raisers for the Republican side in the Spanish Civil War. In addition his wife, Kitty, was a communist, and both were accused during the McCarthy era of having Soviet sympathies. Oppenheimer eventually lost his security clearance; with this development came a loss of political support and eventually a life of obscurity in the Virgin Islands (1). President John F. Kennedy had planned to award him the Enrico Fermi Award but was unfortunately assassinated before he could do so. It was left to President Lyndon Johnson to make the presentation 'for contributions to theoretical physics as a teacher and originator of ideas, and for leadership of the Los Alamos Laboratory and the atomic energy programme during critical years'. As the great rocket scientist Werner von Braun was quoted as saying, 'In England, Oppenheimer would have been knighted' (1). Oppenheimer died of throat cancer in 1967.

War and medicine

It is an awful irony that the destruction of human life caused by the dropping of the atomic bombs on Hiroshima and Nagasaki in 1945 initiated a marvellous set of biological discoveries. A new era of biology inadvertently began and a fascinating series of questions and experiments opened a 'Pandora's box'. As with all scientific discoveries, many people were involved. Only a few names, however, remain in the 'canon'; so these will be mentioned here, although there were many other contributors.

Jacob Bronowski (1908–74), a physicist who is perhaps best remembered as the writer and presenter of the BBC television documentary series *The Ascent of Man*, and Leó Szilárd (1898–1964), a physicist from Budapest, Hungary, who worked on the Manhattan Project, both converted to the study of biology as a result of the devastation the atomic bomb caused in Japan. Egon Lorenz, a physicist who had come to the United States in the 1930s from Germany and had been involved with the Manhattan Project, conducting experiments on the effects of low-dose irradiation on mammals, continued his work after the war at the National Institutes for Health (NIH) laboratories at Bethesda, MD. His experiments, together with those of Leon Orris Jacobson (3), a physician who had also been active in the Manhattan Project, were to change the world of haematology forever.

However, the compartmentalization of scientific knowledge continues to fascinate me. I recently spoke with a retired nuclear scientist in Italy who had lectured in Princeton University and knew Oppenheimer. He said there had been virtually no communication between the biologists interested in the effects of ionizing radiation, and the physicists working on the Manhattan Project. He was completely unaware of the biological experiments of Lorenz and did not know about the stimulus that the atomic bomb had given to the development of bone marrow transplantation.

Of Mice and Men (title of a novel by John Steinbeck, written in 1937)

Most of us receive postcards from friends or relatives while on holiday. The information is usually trivial and related to the place being visited, with remarks such as 'Having a great time! Wish you were here' or some other superficial comment. However, while on holiday in 1950, Lorenz sent quite a different postcard from Windermere, UK to his laboratory assistant, Delta Uphoff; this postcard contained a very special message. In it, he suggested that Uphoff should inject suspensions of normal bone marrow into irradiated mice in order to repopulate their destroyed bone marrow. By the time Lorenz returned to the United States, Uphoff had completed his experiment, and the worlds of biology and medicine were about to change forever: stem cells from one mouse could repopulate the bone marrow of another mouse and give rise to all the blood cells in the recipient. This finding was the first evidence that transplantation of stem cells was possible.

But how could you know a transplant had taken place? Because males and females have different sex chromosomes, the origin of the transplanted cells could easily be established. Animals which had the blood cells of the donor were called 'radiation chimaeras', after the mythical Greek fire-breathing monster, offspring of Echidna and Typhon (Figure 6.2).

Like many discoveries, the idea that bone marrow cells from the healthy donor could divide and multiply and produce all the required cells in the recipient was not new. A Russian pathologist, Alexander A. Maximov (1874–1928), originally from Saint Petersburg but who fled to Chicago in 1922, suggested the unitarian theory of haematopoiesis in 1908. He proposed that all blood cells were derived from a common ancestor or precursor cell which he called a stem cell. It took almost 50 years before his theory could be proven (4).

From the laboratory to the clinic

Until recently, it was relatively common for people to eat animal bone marrow, usually from calves, as a nutritional supplement (Figure 6.3). It is probable that the only nutritional value was in the fat, protein, and the iron content. Mehdi Tavassoli

Fig. 6.2 A drawing of a chimaera, by the artist James Cogan. A chimaera is a mythical creature with the head of a lion, the body of a goat, and the tail of a snake. Successfully transplanted laboratory animals were known as radiation chimaeras.

Reproduced by kind permission of James Cogan. Copyright © 2015 James Cogan.

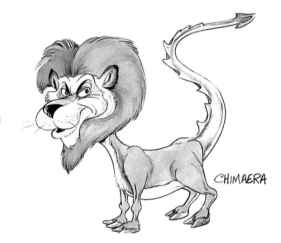

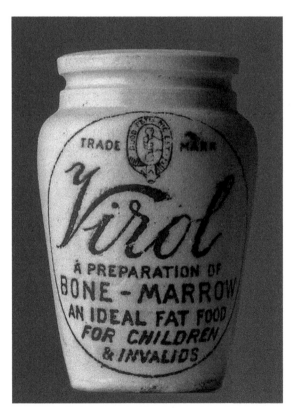

Fig. 6.3 A photograph of a ceramic container used for calf bone marrow. Until the early twentieth century, marrow was valued for its nutritional qualities.

Reproduced by kind permission of Shaun McCann. Copyright © 2015 Shaun McCann.

in his chapter 'Bone Marrow: The Seedbed of Blood' in Wintrobe's book, *Blood, Pure and Eloquent* (5), says: 'From ancient days marrow was used for food and was considered to be rich and nutritious'. However, it was not until the nineteenth century that a German doctor, Franz Ernst Christian Neumann (1834–1918) established the link between bone marrow and blood when in 1868 he wrote: 'The present work intends to demonstrate the physiologic importance of the bone marrow… It operates continuously in a de novo formation of red cells' (5). At the same time, a 22-year-old graduate from the University of Pavia, Giulio Bizzozero (1846–1901), argued that bone marrow was the origin of red and white cells. The theories of Neumann and Bizzozero were vigorously challenged by the 'haematology establishment', and the French doyen of haematology, Georges Hayem (1841–1933), wrote a book repudiating the theories of Bizzozero (5). The concept of stem cells only became fully elaborated with the emergence of nuclear physics.

Serendipity, however, also played a major role in the stem cell story, as it has done over time in many medical and scientific discoveries. In 1958 six laboratory workers in Belgrade were accidentally exposed to ionizing radiation. This accident provided an opportunity to test the 'stem cell' theory. The laboratory workers were sent to George Mathé in Paris; he treated one of them with stem cells from a fetus and subsequently with bone marrow cells from an unrelated volunteer. Unfortunately the interventions were not successful, and the patient died from bleeding. Mathé proceeded to give bone marrow cells to the four remaining patients; happily, two of them eventually recovered normal blood counts, although it was not clear what contribution the transplanted stem cells had made to their recovery; the world still needed large-scale studies to assess the real value of stem cell transplantation and its potential role in treating leukaemia (6, 7). Nonetheless, A. John Barrett, President of the American Society for Blood and Marrow Transplantation in 2010, stated that Georges Mathé should have shared the Nobel Prize awarded to E. Donal Thomas and Joseph E. Murray for their work in transplantation.

Numerous laboratory experiments paved the way for stem cell transplantation, including the identification of 'runt disease', later called 'graft-versus-host disease', in rodents (8, 9), and the identification of the human leucocyte antigen (HLA). However, the individual who gained the world's accolades for clinical bone marrow transplantation was a quiet, retiring, but persistent physician, E. Donal Thomas. He and his team worked relentlessly, initially with hopeless results: the first 200 stem cell transplants they tried failed (10). Yet, Thomas and his team persisted. In time, they moved to a purpose-built hospital in Seattle, WA, at the Fred Hutchinson Cancer Research Center, where they recruited excellent scientific and medical staff; eventually, they had success in 1975 (11). The publication of two seminal papers in 1979 demonstrated the success of bone marrow transplantation in the treatment of leukaemia (12, 13). The demonstration that transplantation of human stem cells could be used to treat leukaemia stimulated widespread interest, and stem cell transplant units were established worldwide. In 1990, Thomas shared the Nobel Prize for Medicine or Physiology with Murray for his contribution to organ transplantation.

Stem cell transplantation

In stem cell transplantation, stem cells are collected from the donor by sticking large needles in the donor's pelvic bones, under general anaesthesia, and removing approximately 1 l of marrow. The number of stem cells required for a successful transplant in humans is the same as in the mouse, adjusted for body size (2×10^8/kg). Following collection from the donor, stem cells are transfused into a large vein in the patient. Then, the waiting begins. Chemicals released by specialized cells in the recipient's bone marrow attract transplanted donor cells. After 14–21 days, the donated stem cells begin to divide and give rise to different types of blood cells. These new blood cells are released into the patient's bloodstream, where they can be counted. Their origin is confirmed by comparing the DNA patterns in donor and patient cells (Figure 6.4).

In the early days of stem cell transplantation, a number of important and forward-looking decisions were made. In the United States, a bone marrow

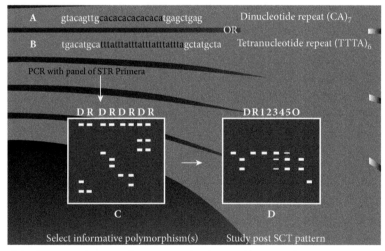

Fig. 6.4 Differences between humans can be detected by DNA size patterns, even if the subjects are of the same sex. A number of techniques are available for analysing DNA. This figure illustrates the use of short tandem sequence repeats to distinguish between donor and host following the amplification of DNA by PCR.

transplant registry was initiated at the University of Milwaukee, WI, in 1972; in Europe, a group of like-minded physicians and scientists, led by Bruno Speck from Switzerland, got together in 1973 to form the European Society for Blood and Marrow Transplantation (EBMT), the main focus of which was to encourage discussion and share findings among stem cell 'transplanters'. The EBMT has been so successful that it now has more than 500 teams from 50 countries reporting data. The National Marrow Donor Program was formed by the US Navy in 1986, followed by establishment in 2004 of the Centre for International Blood and Marrow Transplant Research, which collates data on stem cell transplants performed worldwide.

Stem cell transplantation, unfortunately, is not always successful because of the new man-made disease, graft-versus-host disease, a condition that can be considered the inverse of graft rejection. Immunological cells produced by the transplanted bone marrow cells may recognize minor antigenic differences between the donor and the recipient and thus attack recipient tissue, causing illness of varying severity and that is occasionally fatal. The drugs cyclosporine and methotrexate are given to the recipient to prevent graft-versus-host disease but unfortunately this treatment is not always successful.

Because of this problem, belief persisted that stem cell transplantation from a compatible brother or sister offered the best chance of success. However, over time it became apparent that it was also possible to find suitable donors who were not related to the patient. A world 'club' developed as a result of this discovery, and eventually millions of volunteers had their tissue type measured and entered in a computerized registry (14). This registry is a wonderful example of human altruism and reflects the efforts of doctors, laboratory scientists, and lay organizers. In spite of the logistical and regulatory problems of transporting stem cells from one jurisdiction to another, the procedure has been remarkably successful.

The development of DNA technology is another advance that has revealed many unexpected minor differences in HLA types between individuals who, on preliminary examination, appeared to be identical. Technological advances in HLA typing can, however, be a 'double-edged' sword: although they improve the 'matching' and outcome of unrelated stem cell transplants, they exclude potential donors who would have been considered 'a match' with the use of older and less sensitive methods.

Long-term toxicity in stem cell transplantation

In spite of the success of stem cell transplantation, long-term survivors may encounter numerous problems. Chronic graft-versus-host disease remains a problem, with no great improvements in response to treatment apart from the use of corticosteroids. Many of the long-term problems are related to chronic graft-versus-host disease and the myeloablative conditioning regimens (chemotherapy or irradiation; given to kill off the recipient's bone marrow cells) used prior to transplant. Respiratory complications usually appear within the first 2 years and have a poor outcome. Renal toxicity is usually seen within the first 10 years, and cardiovascular complications usually occur more than 10 years following transplantation. Other complications include cataracts, infertility, endocrine dysfunction, bone and joint complications, and secondary cancers (15). Most stem cell transplant units continue to monitor survivors indefinitely. A rather unusual event, and one that is probably under-reported, is the occurrence of leukaemia in donor cells after transplantation. Such a result suggests that there may be a micro-environmental defect in the marrow stroma in some patients (16–18).

Non-myeloablative stem cell transplants

In order to minimize toxicity and increase the age at which transplantation could be offered, methods of conditioning without resorting to the complete ablation of the recipient's marrow have been investigated. Such preparative or conditioning regimens depend on the use of potent immunosuppression of the recipient together with so-called reduced-intensity conditioning (19). Recently the use of so-called haplo-identical donors (donors who share 50% of the HLA antigens of the recipient), a technique pioneered at Johns Hopkins University in Baltimore, MD, has widened the availability of potential donors. Initial results are promising but long-term follow-up is awaited (20).

Sources of stem cells

Bone marrow, however, is not the exclusive home of stem cells. They are also found in peripheral blood in small numbers and they can be 'mobilized' from bone marrow into the bloodstream by daily injections of recombinant human granulocyte colony-stimulating factor and can thus be collected with the use of a specialized centrifuge. Stem cells also circulate in the blood in large numbers after chemotherapy and thus can be collected for 'autografting'.

Stem cells are also present in the placenta, where they may be found in larger numbers than in peripheral blood (Figure 6.5). Some animals eat the placenta after giving birth and, although there are those who advocate that human mothers should do likewise, this is an unwelcome prescription for the vast majority of women. Another strange use of human placentas is in make-up, by the cosmetic industry, which has also used bull semen and chicken bone marrow in the

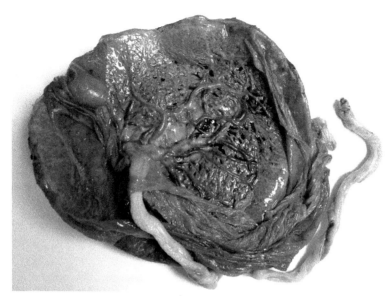

Fig. 6.5 Photograph of a human placenta.

Reproduced by kind permission by Professor John O'Leary. Copyright © 2015 John O'Leary.

manufacture of 'beauty products'. Dried placenta has also been put into cap-sules, as some people believe it contains medicinal properties. However, besides these interesting uses, placental blood is a rich source of stem cells which can be frozen for transplantation at a later date.

The umbilical cord is another source of stem cells. In a private meeting in 1982, Edward A. Boyse, Judith Bard, and Hal Broxmeyer discussed the possibil-ity of using stem cells derived from umbilical cord blood for transplantation; their discussions led to the formation in 1985 of the Biocyte Corporation, whose research demonstrated that stem cells from the placenta and the umbili-cal cord could be used in place of bone marrow in stem cell transplantation (21, 22). Following a number of animal experiments which demonstrated the prolif-erative capacity of stem cells from umbilical cord blood, the stage was set for human transplantation. In 1989 a 5-year-old child with a congenital form of severe anaemia required a stem cell transplant but had no brothers or sisters. The parents had a second child in the hope that he or she would be a 'match' and, indeed, this was the case. Blood removed from umbilical cord after birth was frozen and then used successfully in what was the first umbilical cord stem cell transplant. Although the transplant took place in Paris, the basic laboratory work was done in the United States. The recipient, now in his mid-twenties, is alive and well (23).

One issue concerning umbilical cord blood transplants is that the volumes of cells obtained from umbilical cord blood, and therefore the number of stem cells, are small and usually suited to paediatric transplants. Using two cords or expanding stem cell numbers may be beneficial, and direct intra-bone injection may be better than intravenous injection; however, immune reconstitution and graft rejection remain problems. Improving HLA typing and matching between umbilical cord blood and recipient may also improve the outcome (24). Another, more controversial issue is the long-term storage of umbilical cord blood from healthy babies, as this blood can be frozen at birth for future use. Parents can pay for long-term storage in most countries; however, because of the costs involved, the majority of individuals are excluded from taking part. Therefore, many people believe that umbilical cord should be donated in an altruistic fashion, like blood transfusion.

In spite of these issues, as of 2013, 30,000 umbilical cord blood transplants have been reported. However, the number of such transplants appears to be decreasing, possibly because of the success of haplo-identical transplants (25).

Stem cell transplantation for diseases other than leukaemia

Stem cell transplantation can also be used for the treatment of benign diseases of red cells, namely, sickle cell disease (26), and thalassaemia (27). In these diseases, affected children either make abnormal haemoglobin or cannot make adequate amounts of normal adult haemoglobin. In their severe forms, the diseases result in death during the teenage years or severe complications, such as strokes, in childhood. There are many forms of treatment for these children, including blood transfusion and certain drugs, but none of these interventions provide a cure. Although stem cell transplantation is effective in these disorders, affected people often live in countries with poorly developed health services; thus, the availability of the treatment is severely limited. Stem cell transplants can also be successfully used for the treatment of HIV/AIDS, but the same limitations apply (28, 29).

The use of stems cells is not confined to the treatment of blood diseases. In certain clinical situations, stem cells can be collected, frozen, and subsequently used to rescue patients after large doses of chemotherapy, in so-called autologous transplantation. Many patients become long-term, disease-free survivors after such treatments, and recent evidence suggests that autologous stem cell transplantation may have a role in the treatment of multiple sclerosis (30).

In addition, it also now seems that stem cells in the bone marrow can be made to grow into cells other than blood cells. Under laboratory conditions, these cells may differentiate into heart, muscle, or cartilage. This phenomenon is called 'stem cell plasticity'. Diseases for which the use of stem cell transplantation is being investigated include diabetes mellitus, cerebral palsy, and degenerative diseases of blood vessels in the eye. Whether stem cell therapy will prove beneficial in the long term is still an open question. Clinical trials are continuing, with particular interest focused on cardiac and musculoskeletal diseases.

Induced pluripotent stem cells

Research is also taking place into another type of stem cell. Until recently, it was believed that, when cells undergo a pathway of development or differentiation, this process is irreversible. It now seems that cells which have undergone degrees of differentiation may be made to revert and regain their property of self-renewal. These cells are called induced pluripotent stem cells. Many laboratories are pursuing strategies to understand and utilize pluripotent stem cells, and the NIH Center for Regenerative Medicine is pursuing a research strategy to define the role of pluripotent stem cells. Transplanting pluripotent stem cells would offer patients the possibility of using their own cells and thus avoiding the immune problems associated with allogeneic stem cells. Therapy for age-related macular degeneration is a current focus of attention for the use of pluripotent stem cells clinically (31).

Should the donation of bone marrow and mobilized peripheral blood stem cells be an altruistic act?

In 2012 a disturbing legal judgement was brought to the attention of the haematological community by I. Glenn Cohen (32). Cohen pointed out that the US Court of Appeals for the Ninth Circuit held that the ban on selling bone marrow does not apply to 'peripheral blood stem cells'. This ruling meant that the sale of stem cells for transplantation was now permissible. The court apparently based its opinion on the National Organ Transplant Act. The sale of bone marrow had been prohibited in the United States because it was feared that, if it were permitted, humans would be turned into commodities, the poor might be coerced into selling marrow, the rich would be at an advantage to the poor in terms of finding donors, donors might provide an inaccurate medical history, and financial incentives would reduce altruistic donation and therefore reduce the numbers of voluntary donations. This ruling rang alarm bells in certain communities.

The European Haematology Association responded with an online letter (33) and the Europdonor Foundation, in association with the National Marrow Donor Program (based in the United States), and centres in Europe, Australia, and Taiwan had already outlined the World Marrow Donor Association's views (14) that donation should always be altruistic and that there was no difference between stem cells obtained from peripheral blood and those obtained from bone marrow. Altruism (a term coined by the philosopher Auguste Comte in the nineteenth century) is defined as a concern for others, and a motivation to provide something of value to a party who must be anyone but oneself. Titmuss would be pleased.

Conclusion

No doubt the scientists and doctors who perfected the technique of stem cell transplantation thought this intervention was something new, a novel break-through in medical techniques. This was my view as well, until a colleague placed a translation of *The Táin* on my desk one day (34). *An Táin Bó Cuailgne* is the centrepiece of the eighth-century epic Ulster cycle of heroic Irish tales. It tells the story of a cattle raid by the armies of Queen Medb (Maeve) and King Ailill when they attempted to steal the great Brown Bull of Cuailgne. You can imagine my amazement when I came across the following passage:

> Thereupon Fingin the prophetic leech asked of Cuchulain a vat of marrow wherewith to heal and to cure Cethern son of Fintan. Cuchulain proceeded to the camp and

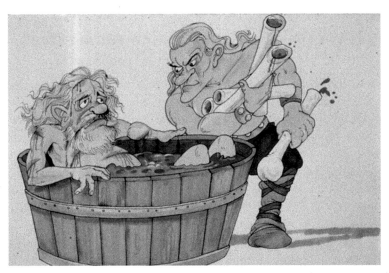

Fig. 6.6 A drawing by the artist James Cogan, showing Cethern in the marrow-mash.

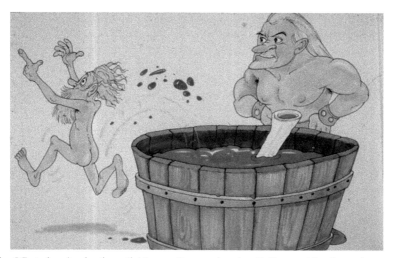

Fig. 6.7 A drawing by the artist James Cogan, showing Cethern arising from the marrow-mash 'after three days and three nights'.

Reproduced by kind permission of the artist, James Cogan. Copyright © 2015 James Cogan.

entrenchment of the men of Erin, and whatsoever he found of herds and flocks and droves there he took away with him. And he made a marrow-mash of their flesh and their bones and their skins; and Cethern son of Fintan was placed in the marrow-bath till the end of three days and three nights (Figure 6.6). And his flesh began to drink in the marrow-bath about him and the marrow-bath entered in within his stabs and his cuts, his sores and his many wounds.

Thereafter he arose from the marrow-bath at the end of three days and three nights. . . . It was thus Cethern arose, with a slab of the chariot pressed to his belly so that his entrails and bowels would not drop out of him' (Figure 6.7).

Although it is not clear how successful the procedure was, nonetheless I realized that I was reading a description of a bone marrow transplantation (albeit xenotransplantation) and was being taught, yet again, that there is nothing totally new under the sun!

References

1 Monk, R. Inside the Centre: The Life of J. Robert Oppenheimer. Anchor Books, New York, NY, 2012.

2 Jungk R. Brighter than a Thousand Suns: A Personal History of the Atomic Scientists. Houghton Mifflin Harcourt, Boston, MA, 1970.

3 Jacobson LO, Marks EK, Robson MJ, Gaston EO, Zirkle ZO. Effect of spleen protection on mortality following x-irradiation. Journal of Laboratory and Clinical Medicine **34**: 1538–43. 1949.

4 **Konstantmov E**. In search of Alexander A. Maximov: The man behind the unitarian theory of hematopoiesis. Perspectives in Biology and Medicine **43** (2): 267–76. 2000.

5 **Wintrobe MW, ed**. Blood, Pure and Eloquent. McGraw-Hill, Inc., New York, NY, 1980.

6 **Mathé G, Bernard J, Schwarzenberg L, Larrieu MJ, Lalanne CM, Dutreix A, et al**. Essai de traitement de sujets atteints de leucemie aigue en remission par irradiation totale suivie de transfusion de moelle osseuse homologue. Revue Francaise D'Etudes Cliniques Et Biologiques **4** (7): 871–5. 1959.

7 **Hakim NS, Papalois VE, eds**. History of Organ and cell transplantation. Imperial College Press, London, 2003.

8 **Van Bekkum DW, De Vries MJ**. Radiation Chimeras. Logos Press, London, 1967.

9 **Bellingham RE, Brent L**. Quantitative studies on tissue transplantation immunity. IV. Induction of tolerance in newborn mice and studies on the phenomenon of runt disease. Philosophical Transactions of the Royal Society of London. Series B. Biological Sciences **242** (694): 439–77. 1959.

10 **Bortin MM**. A compendium of reported human bone marrow transplants. Transplantation **9**: 571–587. 1970.

11 **Thomas ED, Storb R, Clift RA**. Fefer A, Johnson FL, Neiman PE, et al. Bone marrow transplantation. New England Journal of Medicine **292** (17): 832–43. 1975.

12 **Thomas ED, Buckner CD, Clift RA, Fefer A, Johnson FL, Neiman PE, et al**. Marrow transplantation for acute nonlymphocytic leukemia in first remission. New England Journal of Medicine **301** (11): 597–9. 1979.

13 **Thomas ED, Sanders JE, Flournoy N, Johnson FL, Buckner CD, Clift RA, et al**. Marrow transplantation for patients with acute lymphoblastic leukemia in remission. Blood **54** (2): 468–76. 1979.

14 **Boo M, van Walraven SM, Chapman J, Lindberg B, Schmidt AH, Shaw BE, et al**. Remuneration of hematopoietic stem cell donors: Principles and perspective of the World Marrow Association. Blood **117** (1): 21–5. 2010.

15 **Appelbaum FR, Forman SJ, Negrin RS, Blume KG, eds**. Thomas' Hemopoietic Cell Transplantation: Stem Cell Transplantation. Fourth edition. John Wiley & Sons, Hoboken, NJ, 2009.

16 **Browne PV, Lawler MP, McCann SR**. Donor-cell leukemia after bone marrow transplantation for severe aplastic anemia. New England Journal of Medicine **325** (10): 710–13. 1991.

17 **McCann S, Wright E**. Donor cell leukaemia: Perhaps a more common occurrence than we thought! Bone Marrow Transplantation **32** (5): 455–7. 2003.

18 **Hertenstein B, Hambach L, Bacigalupo A, Schmitz N, McCann S, Slavin S, et al**. Development of leukemia in donor cells after allogeneic stem cell transplantation: A survey of the European Society for Blood and Marrow Transplantation (EBMT). Haematologica **90** (7): 669–75. 2005.

19 **Antin JH**. Reduced-intensity stem cell transplantation. ASH Education Program Book **2007** (1): 47–54. 2007.

20 **Luznik L, O'Donnell PV, Symons HJ, Chen AR, Leffell MS, Zahurak M, et al**. HLA-haploidentical bone marrow transplantation for haematological malignancies using

nonmyeloablative conditioning and high-dose, posttransplantation cyclophosphamide. Biology of Blood and Bone Marrow Transplantation **14** (6): 641–50. 2008.

21 **Ballen KK, Gluckman E, Broxmeyer HE**. Umbilical cord transplantation: The first 25 years and beyond. Blood **122** (4): 491–8. 2013.

22 **Broxmeyer HE, Douglas GW, Hangoc G, Cooper S, Bard J, English D, et al**. Human umbilical cord as a potential source of transplantable hematopoietic stem/progenitor cells. Proceedings of the National Academy of Sciences of the United States of America **86** (10): 3828–32. 1989.

23 **Gluckman E, Broxmeyer HA, Auerbach AD, Friedman HS, Douglas GW, Devergie A, et al**. Hematopoietic reconstitution in a patient with Fanconi's anemia by means of umbilical-cord blood from an HLA-identical sibling. New England Journal of Medicine **321**: (17) 1174–8. 1989.

24 **Eapen M, Klein JP, Sanz GF, Spellman S, Ruggeri A, Anasetti C, et al**. Effect of donor-recipient HLA matching at HLA A, B, C and DRB1 on outcomes after umbilical-cord transplantation for leukemia and myelodysplastic syndrome. Lancet Oncology **12** (13): 1214–21. 2011.

25 **Passweg JR, Baldomero H, Bader P, Bonini C, Cesaro S, Dreger P, et al**. Hemopoietic SCT in Europe 2013: Recent trends in the use of alternative donors showing more haploidentical donors but fewer cord blood transplants. Bone Marrow Transplantation **50** (4): 476–82. 2015.

26 **Freed J, Telano J, Small T, Ricci A, Cairo MS**. Allogeneic cellular and autologous stem cell transplantation for sickle cell disease: 'Whom, when, how'. Bone Marrow Transplantation **47** (**12**): 1489–98. 2011.

27 **Angelucci E**. Hematopoietic stem cell transplantation in thalassemia. ASH Education Program Book **2010** (**1**): 456–62. 2010.

28 **Allens K, Hütter G, Hofmann J, Loddenkemper C, Rieger K, Thiel E, et al**. Evidence for the cure of HIV infection by CCR5Δ/Δ32 stem cell transplantation. Blood **117** (10): 2791–9. 2011.

29 **Nathwani N**. Hematopoietic stem cell transplantation in HIV infected patients, in SK Saxena, ed., Current Perspectives in HIV Infection. InTech, Rijeka, 2013, pp. 57–74.

30 **Nash RA, Hutton GJ, Racke MK, Popat U, Devine SM, Griffith LM, et al**. High-dose immunosuppressive therapy and autologous hematopoietic cell transplantation for relapsing-remitting multiple sclerosis (HALT-MS): A 3-year interim report. Journal of the American Medical Association Neurology **72** (2): 159–69. 2015.

31 **O'Brien T, Barry FP**. Stem cell therapy and regenerative medicine. Mayo Clinic Proceedings **84** (10): 859–81. 2009.

32 **Cohen IG**. Selling bone marrow: *Flynn v. Holder*. New England Journal of Medicine **366** (4): 296–7. 2012.

33 **McCann S**. Would you sell peripheral blood derived stem cells? http://www.ehaweb. org/news-room/eha-news article17, 2012.

34 **An Táin Bó Cuailgne**. Translated by Joseph Dunn. Project Gutenberg. (Ebook#16464). 2005.

Chapter 7

Leukaemia

Introduction

The word leukaemia still is associated with foreboding and a fear of premature death. Steady advances have been made in the treatment of childhood leukaemia but, with notable exceptions, the same in not true in adults. The so-called genetic/molecular revolution has extended our understanding of the pathogenesis of many forms of leukaemia but, as yet, has rarely facilitated cure. Chronic myeloid leukaemia is the obvious exception but we wait eagerly to see if the cytogenetic/molecular revolution can provide cures for many elderly patients with leukaemia, as such patients respond poorly to chemotherapy.

Have we a cure?

Unlike many diseases, leukaemia was not really recognized as a distinct entity until early in the nineteenth century. The development of microscopy and subsequently of aniline dyes for staining blood and marrow films made a major contribution to diagnosis and classification of leukaemias. Cytogenetics, immunology, and latterly molecular biology have all contributed to our understanding and treatment of these diseases. However, the word 'leukaemia' still provokes a reaction of horror in the general population, including in some doctors. It is true that the treatment of childhood acute lymphoblastic leukaemia has been a major success story and that the use of tyrosine kinase inhibitors has radically altered the outcome for patients with chronic myeloid leukaemia. The use of all-trans retinoic acid (ATRA) and the old drug arsenic trioxide (As_2O_3) resulted in the cure of many patients with acute promyelocytic leukaemia and through stem cell transplantation, in spite of costs and complications; hope was given to many patients with an otherwise incurable disease. Notwithstanding advances in acute lymphoblastic leukaemia, leukaemia remains a disease of the young and, although mechanisms of the disease are being unravelled, we do not know its cause in most patients. None of the above approaches, except for tyrosine kinase inhibitors, would have been successful without the development of good supportive care with red cell and platelet transfusions, antibiotics, and antifungal therapy.

Who diagnosed leukaemia first?

The book *Leukemia* provides a thorough account of the doctors and scientists involved in the early diagnosis of this group of blood diseases (1). Alfred Armand Louis Marie Velpeau (1795–1867), Rudolf Ludwig Karl Virchow (1821–1902), Bennett, and David Cragie (1793–1866) are all mentioned but, to my mind, Alfred François Donné (1801–78) stands out as a major figure. Donné, who had graduated in Paris in 1831, provided the first description of leukaemia in the *Cours de microscopie* in 1844 when he reported the case of the patient Rayer in Hôpital de la Charité:

> [I found] no trace of purulent matter, neither in the vessels nor in the blood clot. Since I have frequently observed similar cases in the blood of individuals without purulent matter, I think that the excess of white blood cells is due to an arrest of differentiation (*arrêt de l'évolution du sang*). According to my theory about the origin and development of blood cells . . . [the] increase of white cells is the consequence of an arrest in differentiation of these intermediate cells (*ne sont que le résultat d'un arrêt de développement de ces particules intermédiaires*)' (2).

As it turned out, Donné was spot on when he determined that leukaemia was the result of failure of differentiation, although it is easy for us now to understand the difficulties in separating infection and pus from malignancy (3). Bennett and Virchow had debated the issue of suppuration and leukaemia but, unfortunately, Donné was excluded from these discussions as he was not a professor (4). It's amazing now silly and counterproductive academic jealousy can be. Donné was ignored by many in the medical profession, although his work with the daguerreotype, an early photographic process invented by Frenchman Louis Daguerre, led to the development of the first photomicroscope.

Neumann, who also had early and progressive ideas about stem cells, is credited with relating leukaemia to changes in the bone marrow; he also contributed the word 'myelogenous' to the lexicon (5). According to *Leukemia*, in 1876, Friedrich Mosler introduced bone marrow puncture (aspiration) as a means of diagnosing leukaemia (1). In the 1950s and 1960s, many people were involved in developing new drugs, with some degree of success. The seminal discovery of Peter Nowell and David Hungerford in 1960 (6, 7) of the first non-random chromosomal abnormality, the so-called Philadelphia chromosome, in patients with chronic myeloid leukaemia opened a new door to our understanding of leukaemia as an acquired chromosomal disorder. It also initiated the race among clinician/scientists that culminated in the use of tyrosine kinase inhibitors in the twenty-first century and changed the lives of thousands of people with chronic myeloid leukaemia.

The US NIH

Institutions which receive government support have played an important part in haematology. The NIH has an exalted reputation for most doctors, especially in the Western world, due to its role in public health. It owes its origin to the Marine Hospital Service (MHS), which was established in 1798 to provide medical care for sailors; for this service, the sailors paid 20 cents per month. By the early 1880s, the MHS began examining immigrants for signs of infectious diseases. The discoveries of Robert Heinrich Herman Koch (1843–1910) and others in Europe describing the microbiological causes of many infectious led to the establishment in 1887 of a one-room laboratory in the Marine Hospital at Stapleton, Staten Island, NY, under the direction of Joseph J. Kinyoun. His laboratory, called the 'Laboratory of Hygiene', was based on existing German facilities. He used a Zeiss microscope to demonstrate the cholera bacillus to colleagues. In 1891 the laboratory moved to Washington, DC, and in 1901 Congress made $35,000 available for a new building to investigate 'infectious and contagious diseases and matters pertinent to public health'. In 1930 the Ransdell Act created the NIH to allow the application of fundamental chemistry to medical research.

The US National Cancer Institute was established in 1937 and became a designated arm of the NIH in 1944. During World War II, the NIH concentrated on the war effort, which include the development of vaccines and a synthetic form of quinine. The budget of the NIH went from $8 million in 1947 to $1 billion by 1966. In 1953 the Warren Grant Magnuson Clinical Center on the campus of the NIH in Bethesda, MD, opened to bring research laboratories closer to clinicians and to pursue clinical trials. Interestingly, the NIH website states that this development 'did not represent a move toward "socialized medicine," which was opposed by most American physicians in the 1950s' (8). Judging by the hostility to attempts by President Barack Obama to introduce new health insurance legislation in 2008–10, it seems as if that position has not radically changed in the twenty-first century. Philanthropists Albert and Mary Lasker were supporters of the NIH, and Mary was particularly influential in expanding its role and budget.

The war on cancer

In 1971 President Richard Nixon signed the National Cancer Act. Although the word 'war' is not used in the legislation, many people associate the passage of the Act as the beginning of the 'war on cancer', at least in the United States. Whether the idea of a war on cancer is an appropriate one is a moot point, if one is to judge the outcomes of other wars waged by the United States since 1971, as these have been anything but successful. The idea of a war on cancer is borne out by the comments made in 2005 by Andrew von Eschenbach, the director of the National Cancer Institute, who said 'we can make the dream —of a world free of pain and suffering and death due to cancer—a reality' (9). However, since 1971, the terminology has become widespread, with *The Financial Times* in May/June 2014 writing about the pharma industries' 'new front in war on cancer'. Yet, the reality is that we do not know the causes of most common cancers, with exceptions such as lung cancer due to cigarette smoking, so that the cure for most cancers remains elusive. The Human Genome Project has increased our understanding of mechanisms involved in cancer but we have not yet reached the stage that Eschenbach predicted. It should be remembered that an 'association' and a 'cause' are two completely different concepts. Many associations have no biological significance, and the cause of most diseases, excluding infections, remains obscure.

Acute leukaemia in childhood: A success story

There is no doubt that the treatment of childhood leukaemia, acute lymphoblastic leukaemia, has been an outstanding success, with over 90% of children in Western countries becoming long-term disease-free survivors. The story began in the 1960s and has been well documented (1, 10, 11). However, a number of issues remain which need to be clarified. It is true that childhood acute lymphoblastic leukaemia was the first cancer to be brought into remission with chemotherapy, that the folic acid antagonist aminopterin was used successfully in 1948 (12), and that glucocorticoids were first used as a single agent in 1949 (13). The initial euphoria, well justified, was tempered when central nervous system (CNS) disease and testicular relapse became evident. CNS prophylaxis was undertaken with cranio/spinal irradiation and later with cranial irradiation and intrathecal methotrexate. Although these modalities were effective, they were also accompanied by significant toxicity. Testicular relapse was initially prevented by irradiation but later it became obvious that testicular leukaemia was a manifestation of generalized disease relapse. CNS leukaemia could be prevented with large doses of methotrexate and intrathecal therapy. Happily now, because of well-conducted clinical trials and research, we can offer a 90% chance of disease-free survival to children with acute lymphoblastic leukaemia without the use of radiotherapy and with minimal toxicity.

Less is more

The main question currently posed is, can some children with acute lymphoblastic leukaemia be cured with 'less' than the present approach and can we

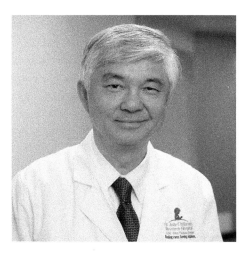

Fig. 7.1 A photograph of Ching-Hon Pui. When I interviewed Pui in a recent podcast, he emphasized how important it was to treat the patient and his/her family and not just the disease.

Reproduced by kind permission of the European Hematology Association and Professor Ching-Hon Pui.

alter therapy to improve the prognosis? Undoubtedly, using molecular techniques to measure the degree of corticosteroid response has made it possible to adjust treatment in certain patients with persistent disease. As Ching-Hon Pui at St Jude Children's Research Hospital said in a recent podcast, 'Yes, for low-risk patients and those in whom the minimal residual disease assay reveals <0.01% leukaemia cells in the bone marrow, then treatment can be less intense and still achieve a >90% long-term cure rate. Whether duration of treatment can be reduced is not clear' (14) (Figure 7.1).

Acute myeloid leukaemia: A disease of the elderly

Acute myeloid leukaemia continues to be a huge problem for patients and doctors. Although great strides have been made in understanding the biology of the disease, the unfortunate fact is that most patients with acute myeloid leukaemia are over 60 years at the time of diagnosis (15). Apparently, age does make a difference and, apart from co-morbidity in the elderly, there may be inherent differences in the response of the leukaemic cells to chemotherapy (15). The recently introduced techniques of molecular biology, genomics, and whole genome sequencing have undoubtedly shed light on disease mechanisms but the cause of acute myeloid leukaemia and effective treatment for the majority of patients still elude us. Increasing doses of chemotherapy with the addition of antibody-directed drugs may improve outcome. The ability to dissect prognostic factors and decide which patients might benefit from allogeneic stem cell transplantation may be helpful (16) but the challenge of successfully treating elderly patients remains.

Genes and acute myeloid leukaemia

Some genetic aberrations, such as t(8;21)/*AML1–ETO* (*RUNX1–RUNX1T1*), inv(16)/*CBFB–MYH2*, or t(15;17)/*PML–RARA*, are associated with specific phenotypes, of which more later. Unravelling the genetics and epigenetics of leukaemogenesis has proven to be complicated. A number of different genetic abnormalities can lead to leukaemia, including mutations that interfere with transcription and thus block cell differentiation, activating mutations that lead to increased cell proliferation, and mutations that affect cell-cycle regulation and apoptosis. To make things even more complicated, different types of mutations may occur within the same leukaemia. Thus, mutations may both cause a block in differentiation and be associated with subsequent mutations resulting in increased cell proliferation. Epigenetic phenomena, such as hypermethylation of DNA, are frequently found in acute myeloid leukaemia; however, although hypomethylating agents and histone deacetylase inhibitors have offered some improvement in blood counts in patients with myelodysplasia, the results of such treatment have been disappointing. Recent techniques such as whole genome sequencing provide further insight into the biology of acute myeloid leukaemia, especially in large numbers of patients who have a normal karyotype (17, 18). However the heterogeneity of the genetic abnormalities in acute myeloid leukaemia has, so far, militated against so-called targeted therapy. Consequently, Gail J. Roboz, Director of the Weill Cornell Leukemia Program, has called for a change in clinical trials for acute myeloid leukaemia so that new agents can be tested on patients in remission, to see if the remission is prolonged, as well as for large cooperative trials for meaningful subgroup analysis based on molecular typing (19).

Personalized treatment/medicine for leukaemia: The story of acute promyelocytic leukaemia

Relevant genetic markers have increased our knowledge of disease mechanisms and 'may' provide guidance for an individualized approach to the treatment of some patients in the ideal setting of a sophisticated hospital environment. Although cytogenetic abnormalities have been identified in 55% of patients with acute myeloid leukaemia, new techniques have uncovered molecular markers in patients in whom the karyotype is reported as normal. The story of acute promyelocytic leukaemia, a variant of acute myeloid leukaemia, is a remarkable development in the treatment of leukaemia.

Acute promyelocytic leukaemia was first described in 1957, when Leif K. Hillested coined the term 'acute promyelocytic leukaemia' for an acute myeloid leukaemia variant that was associated with atypical promyelocytes, hypofibrinogenaemia, and a severe bleeding tendency (20). In 1976 a number of haematologists published a very important paper which outlined the morphological classification of acute leukaemia (21). This so-called FAB (French, British, American) classification recognized acute promyelocytic leukaemia as a distinct morphological entity and, in 1977, Janet D. Rowley and colleagues demonstrated presence of a consistent translocation between Chromosome 15 and 17 (termed t(15;17)) in acute promyelocytic leukaemia cells (22). Although the anthracycline daunorubicin had been used to induce remission in acute promyelocytic leukaemia, a high number of patients treated with this drug had died from uncontrolled bleeding, and overall survival at 5 years remained poor. However, acute promyelocytic leukaemia can now be cured without classic, cytotoxic chemotherapy, with the use of two differentiating agents: ATRA and arsenic trioxide.

ATRA

In 1981 Theodore R. Breitman induced differentiation of human acute promyelocytic leukaemia cells with retinoic acid (23). Christine Chomienne then demonstrated the differentiating effects of ATRA on acute promyelocytic leukaemia cells in vitro and the fact that ATRA was ten times more potent than 13-*cis* retinoic acid. Then, in 1987 Laurent Degos from the INSERM (Institute National de la Santé et de la Recherche Médicale), together with Zhen-Yi Wang of Shanghai Jiao Tong University, witnessed the first treatment of humans with acute promyelocytic leukaemia with ATRA in Shanghai (24). Subsequently, in 1988 a paper appeared in the journal *Blood* from investigators in Shanghai, claiming that remission in acute promyelocytic leukaemia could be induced using the differentiating agent ATRA (25). Wang, together with Zhu Chen, who had been a student of Wang and had worked with Degos at INSERM, explained that, in the days following the Cultural Revolution in China, a search was made for ways of treating malignant diseases other than with chemotherapy (26). This approach may have reflected the practical problems of obtaining chemotherapy and providing supportive care. Although in vitro data on the cellular differentiation potential of retinoic acid were available in China, Europe, and the United States, there appeared to be no reason to use retinoic acid outside China, as acute promyelocytic leukaemia responded fairly well to chemotherapy. The retinoid used by Western countries, 13-*cis* retinoic acid, produced by that the pharmaceutical company Roche, did not work in vivo (27), although its in vitro effect on acute promyelocytic leukaemia cells was similar to that of ATRA (28). Therefore, the patients in the first Western pilot study in 1988 were treated with ATRA produced in China. When diplomatic relations between France and China ceased because of the Tiananmen Square Massacre in June 1989, Roche France helped to produce the ATRA needed to allow patients to continue their treatment. Degos, then at the Memorial Sloan Kettering Cancer Center in New York, also persuaded Roche Nutley in New Jersey to manufacture ATRA (24). The results from the clinical trials led to approval by the FDA and the European Medicines Association (29). The t(15;17) translocation in acute promyelocytic leukaemia was subsequently shown to produce the PML–RAR alpha fusion protein, which inhibits the differentiation of myeloid precursors (30, 31). ATRA overcomes the dominant-negative effect of the PML–RAR alpha fusion protein and induces differentiation of the leukaemia cells, thus allowing patients with acute promyelocytic leukaemia to achieve complete remission (32). ATRA is, however, rapidly metabolized; therefore, complementary chemotherapy is required to sustain complete remission (33).

Arsenic

Traditional treatments may have a 'scientific' basis and should always be investigated. Although arsenic had been used in Manchuria 2000 years ago, it was only first reported as a treatment for leukaemia in the Western literature in 1878; it later became a popular treatment for chronic myeloid leukaemia in the 1930s (34). The compound arsenic trioxide has been under investigation in China as an anticancer treatment since the 1970s; Chinese investigators first reported responses to intravenous arsenic trioxide in patients with acute promyelocytic leukaemia in 1992 (35). Martin S. Tallman and Jessica K. Altman, both at the Robert H. Lurie Comprehensive Cancer Center in Chicago, IL, have stated that the addition of arsenic trioxide 'may replace conventional therapy' (36), and Francesco Lo-Coco at University of Rome, Tor Vergata and colleagues from Gruppo Italiano Malattie Ematologiche dell'Adulto, the German–Austrian Acute Myeloid Leukemia Study Group, and Study Alliance Leukemia have recently shown that a combination of ATRA and arsenic trioxide is at least as good as ATRA combined with chemotherapy at treating low-risk acute promyelocytic leukaemia (white blood cell count $<10 \times 10^9/l$) (37). Thus, both agents now have a definite place in Western medicine in the treatment of acute promyelocytic leukaemia.

Myelodysplastic syndromes

In 2008 the WHO defined myelodysplastic syndromes as a group of clonal disorders occurring in adults of advanced age (median age at presentation is 70 years) and which are characterized by bone marrow hypercellularity and peripheral blood cytopenias (38). Until the late 1970s, these syndromes were simply known in purely descriptive term as 'marrow hypercellularity with peripheral pancytopenia'. Progression of a myelodysplastic syndrome to acute myeloid leukaemia is the natural course in many patients but varies according to subtype. The majority of myelodysplastic syndromes occur without any known cause, although some may be caused by chemotherapy for other malignancies while others, such as Fanconi anaemia, are associated with congenital lesions. In the 1990s, there was an explosion of knowledge regarding genetic and molecular abnormalities associated with myelodysplastic syndromes, and epigenetic abnormalities associated with myelodysplastic syndromes have also been defined. A number of prognostic systems have been published; but, sadly, although low-dose chemotherapy, hypomethylating agents, and histone deacetylase inhibitors have all been tried, the cure for myelodysplastic syndromes remains elusive, and supportive care continues to be the cornerstone of management. Haematopoietic stem cell transplantation, however, may be appropriate for young patients with aggressive disease.

Chronic myeloid leukaemia

The diagnosis of chronic myeloid leukaemia was probably one of the most depressing therapeutic experiences for a haematologist until the early 1980s. Prior to the advent of treatment with tyrosine kinase inhibitors, the diagnosis of chronic myeloid leukaemia was a death sentence unless a suitable donor was available for haematopoietic stem cell transplantation. Symptomatic control was relatively easy but, as the disease progressed, premature death became inevitable. Disease progression was not always easy to predict but the knowledge of premature death hung over the patient like the sword of Damocles.

Patients presented with night sweats and fatigue, and the diagnosis was relatively easily made by the finding of an enlarged spleen and an elevated white cell count with premature white cell precursors in the peripheral blood. Finding the Philadelphia chromosome was a major breakthrough (6). The discovery by Rowley that the Philadelphia chromosome resulted from a reciprocal exchange between the long arms of Chromosomes 9 and 22 opened the door to understanding the biology of chronic myeloid leukaemia and culminated in effective treatment (39).

Imatinib: The magic bullet

The story of the development of imatinib brings together basic research into oncogenes, viral oncogenesis, and the observation that the fusion protein BCR–ABL was the cause of the malignant phenotype in chronic myeloid leukaemia. The important link between a determined scientist, Joerg Zimmerman at Ciba–Geigy (now Novartis) and a haematologist at the Oregon Health and Science University, Brian J. Druker, was at the heart of the development of tyrosine kinase inhibitors, and Druker's name is now firmly linked to the use of tyrosine kinase inhibitors for this disease. Brian is a mild-mannered man; in a recent review of his work, he recalled how 'at one time I was told I had no future' (40). In that same review, he points out how seminal and sometimes apparently unconnected pieces of research eventually resulted in the clinical and very successful use of imatinib, the first tyrosine kinase inhibitor. The first presentation of the inhibition of chronic myeloid leukaemia colony formation and suppression of BCR–ABL-expressing cells in vitro at the annual meeting of the American Society of Hematology in 1998 was attended by about 50 people (in contrast, congress attendance comprised about 20,000 delegates). Following this presentation, Druker formed a team of investigators, including John Goldman, Charles Sawyers, and Moshe Talpaz. However, in spite of this formidable team, it took a lot of persuasion to get the pharmaceutical company Novartis to produce enough drug to conduct meaningful clinical trials on a relatively rare disease, particularly when a compound that the company thought would never work was being used. As Druker said in his review, it was also important to persuade Novartis that they could recoup their investment in the treatment of an uncommon disease. At €30,000 per year per patient for a drug that at present is taken for life, the investment was obviously rewarding. The so-called second-generation tyrosine kinase inhibitors are even more expensive; consequently, the widespread use of this class of drugs is problematical for many health services and patients. This problem was highlighted in a multi-authored paper (>100 experts in chronic myeloid leukaemia from North America, Europe, Russia, Latin America, Australia, Asia, the Middle East, and Africa) in *Blood* in 2013 (41).

After imatinib

There is no doubt that imatinib changed the world for patients with chronic myeloid leukaemia. Not only did it bring their spleen size and blood counts back to normal and make the abnormal Philadelphia chromosome disappear with relatively little toxicity, but the drug prevented the disease from progressing to the much-feared 'blast crisis'. In practice, this means that the number of patients with so-called chronic-phase chronic myeloid leukaemia continues to grow; in India, which has a population of 1.2 billion, it is estimated that there will be 120,000 people taking imatinib, at a cost of $3.6 billion. In April 2013 the Supreme Court of India upheld the rejection of the patent application (1602/MAS/1998) filed by Novartis AG for Gleevec/Glivec (imatinib) in 1998 before the Indian Patent Office. A number of generic tyrosine kinase inhibitors are now available in India at a cost of $50–$100 per month, or $72 million for 120,000 patients. Novartis has since launched a drive to assist patients who could not afford Gleevec/Glivec and, at the time of publication, roughly 16,000 people receive Gleevec/Glivec free of charge.

Treating with, monitoring, and stopping tyrosine kinase inhibitors in patients with chronic myeloid leukaemia

The number of patients receiving haematopoietic stem cell transplantation has decreased markedly in most registries (Figure 7.2), owing to the success of treatment with tyrosine kinase inhibitors. Very few, if any, patients now require haematopoietic stem cell transplantation at the time of diagnosis of their chronic myeloid leukaemia. An editorial in *Acta Haematologica* in 2013 by Robert P. Gale and John M. Goldman suggested that stem cell transplants should only be offered to patients who don't respond to tyrosine kinase inhibitors, have a problem with drug compliance, or show evidence of disease progression in spite of tyrosine kinase inhibitor therapy (42).

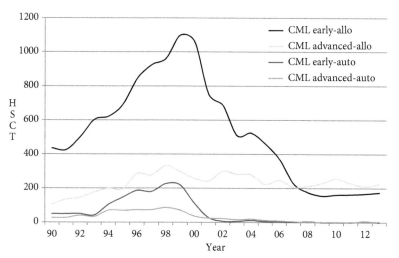

Fig. 7.2 The numbers of patients receiving haemopoietic stem cell transplantation for chronic myeloid leukaemia, from 1990 to 2012. Patients receiving allogeneic haematopoietic cell transplantation at an early stage of the disease are designated 'CML early-allo'; patients receiving allogeneic haematopoietic cell transplantation at an advanced stage of the disease are designated 'CML advanced-allo'; patients receiving autologous haematopoietic cell transplantation at an early stage of the disease are designated 'CML early-auto'; and those receiving autologous haematopoietic cell transplantation at an early stage of the disease are designated 'CML late-auto'; HSCT, haematopoietic stem cell transplantation.

We can now monitor the patient's response to tyrosine kinase inhibitors in a number of ways, including blood counts, spleen size, karyotyping, fluorescent in situ hybridization analysis, and measurement of BCR–ABL1 transcripts. Although the second-generation tyrosine kinase inhibitors lead to a more rapid and deeper molecular response than the first-generation ones, there is no evidence yet that they offer any survival advantage. In addition, they are more expensive and more toxic than imatinib.

There are a number of reasons why a patient might lose his/her response to imatinib. One of these came as a surprise to many physicians: poor compliance (43). Measurement of plasma imatinib levels was suggested as a way of detecting compliance failures (44); however, it was found that patients may take the drug a few days before the clinic visit and in order to have plasma levels within the therapeutic range for the duration of the test (44). The issue persists, and the reasons for non-compliance are in urgent need of additional study.

When to stop tyrosine kinase inhibitors?

In a beautifully written editorial in 2013, Gale and Goldman make the point that, although a complete cytogenetic response is desirable, molecular responses are still awaiting prospective clinical trials to validate their importance in outcome (42). Most investigators believe that a reduction in BCR–ABL1 transcript levels of <10% at 3 months may be the best predictor of survival. Patterns of rise in BCR–ABL1 transcript levels may indicate the evolution of a resistant clone or a compliance problem (45).

The most vexed question for patients, doctors, and health services is, when can tyrosine kinase inhibitors safely be stopped? Some investigators suggest that observation of a deep molecular response for 2 years may be sufficient to consider stopping tyrosine kinase inhibitors. Yet the problem is, what is a deep molecular response? As François X. Mahon points out, discontinuation of treatment should only be contemplated within the confines of a clinical study (46).

BCR–ABL1 kinase domain mutations in chronic myeloid leukaemia

Loss of response to tyrosine kinase inhibitors can be due to a number of mechanisms, including poor compliance, as mentioned above, or mutations in the ABL1 kinase domain. Many mutations have been documented and the most dreaded is the T315I, which renders the patient resistant to all tyrosine kinase inhibitors except ponatinib, which unfortunately is a toxic agent. The choice of stem cell transplantation or ponatinib for patients with the T315I mutation will depend on the patient's age and the existence of a suitable donor.

Recommendations for the management of chronic myeloid leukaemia have evolved since the introduction of tyrosine kinase inhibitors and were refined in 2013: the ABL1 kinase domain mutations E255K/V, F359C/V, and Y253H are more sensitive to dasatinib than to nilotinib, and F317L and V299L are more sensitive to nilotinib than to dasatinib (47).

Thus, chronic myeloid leukaemia, a disease that was universally fatal 15 years ago, is now eminently, albeit very expensively, treatable, and current clinical issues include compliance and discontinuation of treatment. There is also another question: is chronic myeloid leukaemia a paradigm for cancer, or just a strange disease?

Minimal residual disease in leukaemia

The term coined to describe the concept that disease relapse was due to the re-emergence of small numbers of malignant cells not killed by the initial therapy was 'minimal residual disease', which was first investigated in non-Hodgkin lymphoma and in acute lymphoblastic leukaemia.

In the mid-1980s, interest was generated in the possible use of autologous bone marrow transplantation to cure adult intermediate-grade or high-grade non-Hodgkin lymphoma (48). Subsequently, PCR-based assays indicated that were fewer relapses following autologous transplantation if the bone marrow or mobilized peripheral blood stem cells were free of 'molecular' disease (49).

Acute lymphoblastic leukaemia of childhood has provided a vehicle to explore different methods of identifying residual leukaemia cells after or during treatment (50, 51). Such methods include immunophenotyping or molecular analysis, which may enable clinicians to adjust therapy. As Pui observed in a recent podcast, 'The white blood cell count at diagnosis is no longer of prognostic significance, as treatment can be intensified in this group. The absence of leukaemic cells in the bone marrow by flow cytometry at Day 14 strongly influences treatment schedules' (14).

The cytogenetic abnormality in chronic myeloid leukaemia provided a method for detection of residual disease but measurement proved difficult to standardize and results were very dependent on the number of metaphases counted (52). The identification of the BCR–ABL1 fusion gene facilitated the establishment of a PCR test to detect low levels of the fusion gene transcripts (53, 54). Thus, monitoring of patients with chronic myeloid leukaemia receiving tyrosine kinase inhibitors is now done by molecular analysis of *BCR–ABL1* transcripts (55, 56) although, as Goldman and Gale point out, analysis of the results should take into consideration the methodology and sensitivity of the assay (42).

Chronic lymphocytic leukaemia: The one that got left behind

Although chronic lymphocytic leukaemia, a B-cell disease, is the most common form of leukaemia in the Western world, with a relevant clinical staging defined in the mid-1970s (57, 58), it is only relatively recently that it has entered the 'molecular' age. We now have a number of molecular parameters in addition to clinical signs and symptoms, although the latter are still important for diagnosis. In a recent review, Nicholas Chiorazzi focused on three prognostic indicators: genetic abnormalities, expression of specific proteins, and the immunoglobulin heavy chain variable region (*IGHV*) mutation status (59). Genetic abnormalities include del(13q), Trisomy 12, del(11q), and del(17p). Specific proteins in or on the chronic lymphocytic leukaemia cell surface including CD38 and Zap-70, and the mutational status of *IGHV* are all important. Sometimes, these different abnormalities occur together. For example, del(13q) is usually found in patients with mutated *IGHV*, and these patients appear to have a more favourable outcome compared to those with del(17p) and who have aggressive disease.

For many years, treatment for chronic lymphocytic leukaemia consisted of chlorambucil, fludarabine, or combinations of both, together with mitoxantrone and with or without the monoclonal antibody rituximab. Since 2010, no doubt spurred on by the success of tyrosine kinase inhibitors in chronic myeloid leukaemia, a number of new agents have been investigated, including antibodies, 'engineered' T-cells, tyrosine kinase inhibitors, and mTOR inhibitors. However, as Michael Hallek pointed out in 2013, chronic lymphocytic leukaemia is a biologically complex disease, unlike chronic myeloid leukaemia, which is initiated by a single oncogene (*BCR–ABL1*). He also believes that these 'new' agents will still have to be combined with chemotherapy (60). Interestingly, a number of the new agents are associated with a rise in peripheral blood lymphocyte counts, as occurs with corticosteroids, and this finding may be disturbing to both patients and their doctors. Rather than pursuing a cure at present, it may be that disease control allied to a good quality of life should be the goal.

Conclusion

In summary, there has undoubtedly been great progress in the treatment of leukaemia since the 1940s. Some forms of leukaemia are curable without chemotherapy, and the introduction of so-called targeted therapy with tyrosine kinase inhibitors for chronic myeloid leukaemia has completely changed the prognosis for that disease. Haemopoietic stem cell transplantation, although toxic, expensive, and difficult, still provides a cure for many patients. In spite of all these advances, however, most adults with acute leukaemia or myelodysplastic syndrome are destined to die from their disease, and the causes of these fatal illnesses continue to elude us.

References

1 **Henderson ES, Lister TA, Greaves MF, eds**. Leukemia. Seventh edition. Saunders, Philadelphia, PA, 2002.

2 **Degos L**. Personal communication. 2014.

3 **Degos L, Hirst W, Buggins A, Mufti G, Mercier E, Branger B**. John Hughes Bennett, Rudolph Virchow . . . and Alfred Donné: The first description of leukemia. Hematology Journal **2** (1): 1. 2001.

4 **Diamantis A, Magiorkinis E, Androutsos**. Alfred François Donné (1801–78): A pioneer of microscopy, microbiology and haematology. Journal of Medical Biography **17** (2): 81–7. 2009.

5 **Neumann E**. Ein Fall von Leukämie mit Erkrankung des Knochenmarkes. Archives Heilkunde **11**: 1–14. 1870.

6 **Nowell PC, Hungerford DA**. A minute chromosome human chronic granulocytic leukemia. Science **132** (3438): 1497. 1960.

7 **Nowell PC, Hungerford DA**. Chromosome studies in human leukemia: Chronic granulocytic leukemia. Journal of the National Cancer Institute **27** (5): 1013. 1961.

8 **Office of NIH History**. A Short History of the National Institutes of Health. https://history.nih.gov/exhibits/history/docs/page_08.html. Accessed 14 Oct 2015.

9 **Eschenbach A von**. Eliminating the suffering and death due to cancer by 2015. Medical Progress Bulletin, Manhattan Policy Institute **1**: http://www.manhattan-institute.org/html/mpb_01.htm. 2005.

10 **Wintrobe MM, ed**. Blood, Pure and Eloquent. McGraw-Hill Inc., New York, NY, 1980.

11 **Inaba H, Greaves M, Mulligan CG**. Acute lymphoblastic leukaemia. Lancet **381** (9881): 1943–55. 2013.

12 **Farber S, Diamond LK, Mercer RD, Sylvester RF Jr, Wolff JA**. Temporary remissions in acute leukemia in children produced by folic acid antagonist 4- aminopteroylglutamic acid (aminopterin). New England Journal of Medicine **238** (23): 787–93. 1948.

13 **Pearson OH, Eliel LP**. Use of pituitary adrenocorticotropic hormone (ACTH) and cortisone in lymphomas and leukemia. Journal of the American Medical Association **144** (16): 1349–53. 1950.

14 **McCann S**. Interview with Ching-Hon Pui on Less is more Is this the way forward in ALL: February 2012 [podcast]. http://www.multiwebcast.com/_ehapodcast/medias/17915_Ching-Hon_Pui.mp3, 2012.

15 **Burnett AK**. Treatment of acute myeloid leukemia: Are we making progress? ASH Education Program Book **2012** (1): 1–6. 2012.

16 **Haferlach T**. Molecular genetic pathways as therapeutic targets in acute myeloid leukemia. ASH Education Program Book **2008** (1): 400–11. 2008.

17 **Welch JS, Link DC**. Genomics of AML: Clinical application of next-generation sequencing. ASH Education Program Book **2011** (1): 30–5. 2011.

18 **Dohner H, Gaidzik VI**. Impact of genetic factors on treatment decisions in AML. ASH Education Program Book **2011** (1): 36–42. 2011.

19 **Roboz GJ**. Novel approaches to the treatment of acute myeloid leukemia. ASH Education Program Book **2011** (1): 43–50. 2011.

20 **Hillested LK**. Acute promyelocytic leukaemia. Acta Medica Scandinavica **159** (3): 189–95. 1957.

21 **Bennett JM, Catovsky D, Daniel MT, Flandrin G, Galton DAG, Gralnick HR, et al**. Proposals for the classification of acute leukaemias. French-British-American (FAB) co-operative group. British Journal of Haematology **33** (4): 451–8. 1976.

22 **Rowley JD, Golomb HM, Dougherty C**. 15/17 Translocation, a consistent chromosomal change in acute promyelocytic leukaemia. Lancet **1** (810): 549–50. 1977.

23 **Breitman TR, Collins AJ, Keene BR**. Terminal differentiation of human promyelocytic leukemia cells in primary culture in response to retinoic acid. Blood **57** (6): 1000–8. 1981.

24 **Degos Laurent**. Personal communication. 2014.

25 **Meng-er H, Yu-chen Y, Shu-rong C, Jin-Ren C, Jia-Xiang L, Lin Z, et al**. Use of all-trans retinoic acid in the treatment of acute promyelocytic leukemia. Blood **72** (2): 567–72. 1988.

26 **Wang ZY, Chen Z**. Acute promyelocytic leukemia: From highly fatal to highly curable. Blood **111** (5): 260–70. 2008.

27 **Chomienne C, Ballerini P, Balintrand N, Amar M, Bernard JF, Boivin P, et al**. Retinoic acid therapy for promyelocytic leukaemia. Lancet **2** (8665): 746–7. 1989.

28 **Chomienne C, Ballerini P, Balintrand N, Daniel MT, Fenaux P, Castaigne S, et al**. All-trans retinoic acid in acute promyelocytic leukemias. II. In vitro studies: Structure-function relationships. Blood **76** (9): 1710–19. 1990.

29 **Chomienne C**. Personal communication. 2014.

30 **de Thè H, Chomienne C, Lanotte M, Degos L, Degean A**. The t(15;17) translocation of acute promyelocytic leukaemia fuse the retinoic receptor α gene with a novel transcribed locus. Nature **347** (6293): 558–61. 1990.

31 **Shen ZX, Chen GQ, Ni JH, Li XS, Xiong SM, Qiu QY, et al**. Use of arsenic trioxide (As_2O_3) in the treatment of acute promyelocytic leukemia (APL): II. Clinical efficacy and pharmacokinetics in relapsed patients. Blood **89** (9): 3354–60. 1997.

32 **Castaigne S, Chomienne C, Daniel MT, et al**. All-trans retinoic acid as a differentiation therapy for acute promyelocytic leukemia. I. Clinical studies. Blood **76** (9): 1704–9. 1990.

33 **Degos L, Wang YZ**. All *trans* retinoic acid in acute promyelocytic leukemia. Oncogene **20** (49): 7140–5. 2001.

34 **Altman KH**. The history of arsenic trioxide in cancer therapy. Oncologist **6** (Suppl 2): 1–2. 2001.

35 **Wang ZY**. Ham Wasserman lecture: Treatment of acute leukemia by inducing differentiation and apoptosis. ASH Education Program Book **2003** (1): 1–13. 2003.

36 **Tallman MS, Altman JK**. How I treat acute promyelocytic leukemia. Blood **114** (25): 5126–35. 2009.

37 **Lo-Coco F, Awisati G, Vignelli M, Thiede C, Orlando SM, Iacobelli S, et al**. Retinoic acid and arsenic trioxide for acute promyelocytic leukemia. New England Journal of Medicine **369** (2): 111–21. 2013.

38 **Brunning RD, Orazi A, Germing U, Le Beau MM**. Myelodysplastic syndromes/neoplasms, overview, in Swerdlow SH, Campo E, Harris NL, Jaffe ES, Pileri SA, Stein H,

et al., WHO Classification of Tumours of Haematopoietic and Lymphoid Tissues. Fourth edition. IARC, Lyon, 2008, pp. 88–93.

39 **Rowley J.** A new consistent abnormality in chronic myelogenous leukemia identified by quinacrine fluorescence and Giemsa staining. Nature **243** (5405): 290–3. 1973.

40 **Druker BJ.** Translation of the Philadelphia chromosome into therapy for CML. Blood **112** (13): 309–18.

41 **Experts in Chronic Myeloid Leukemia.** The price of drugs for chronic myeloid leukemia (CML) is a reflection of the unsustainable prices of cancer drugs: From the perspective of a large group of CML experts. Blood **121** (22): 4439–42. 2013.

42 **Gale RP and Goldman JM.** Treating chronic myeloid leukemia in the era of tyrosine kinase inhibitors. Acta Haematologica **130** (3): 192–5. 2013.

43 **Marin D, Bazeos A, Mahon FX, Eliasson L, Milojkovic D, Bua M, et al.** Adherence is the critical factor for achieving molecular responses in patients with chronic myeloid leukemia who achieve complete cytogenetic responses on imatinib. Leukemia **28** (14): 2381–8. 2010.

44 **Mahon FX, Molimard M.** Correlation between trough plasma concentrations and clinical response in chronic myeloid leukemia. Leukemia Research **33** (8): 1148–9. 2009.

45 **Branford S, Yeung DT, Prime JA, Choi SY, Bang JH, Park JE, et al.** BCR-ABLI doubling times more reliably assess the dynamics of CML relapse compared with the BCR-ABLI fold rise: Implications for monitoring and management. Blood **119** (18): 4264–71. 2012.

46 **Mahon FX, Réa D, Guilhot J, Guilhot F, Huguet F, Nicolini F, et al.** Discontinuation of imatinib in patients with chronic myeloid leukaemia who have maintained complete molecular remission for at least two years: The prospective, multicentre, Stop Imatinib (STIM) trial. Lancet Oncology **11** (11): 1029–35. 2010.

47 **Bacarrani M, Deininger MW, Rosti G, Hochhaus A, Soverini S, Apperley JF, et al.** European Leukemia Net recommendations for the management of chronic myeloid leukemia. Blood **122** (6): 872–84. 2013.

48 **Philip T, Armitage JO, Spitzer G, Chauvin F, Jagannath S, Cahn JY, et al.** High-dose therapy and autologous bone marrow transplantation after failure of conventional chemotherapy in adults with intermediate-grade or high-grade non-Hodgkin's lymphoma. New England Journal of Medicine **316** (24): 1493–8. 1987.

49 **Corradini P, Astolfi M, Cherasco C, Ladetto M, Voena C, Caracciolo D, et al.** Molecular monitoring of minimal residual disease in follicular and mantle cell non-Hodgkin's lymphoma treated with high-dose chemotherapy and peripheral blood progenitor cell autografting. Blood **89** (2): 724–31. 1997.

50 **Ryan J, Quinn F, Meunier A, Boublikova L, Crampe M, Tewari P, et al.** Minimal residual disease detection in childhood acute lymphoblastic leukaemia patients at multiple time-points reveals high levels of concordance between molecular and immunophenotypic approaches. British Journal of Haematology **144** (1): 107–15. 2009.

51 **Øbro NF, Ryder LP, Madsen HO, Andersen MK, Lausen B, Hasle H, et al.** Identification of residual leukemic cells by flow cytometry in childhood B-cell precursor acute lymphoblastic leukemia: Verification of leukemic state by flow-sorting and molecular/cytogenetic methods. Haematologica **97** (1): 137–41. 2012.

52 **Goldman JM, Gale RP.** What does MRD in leukemia really mean? Leukemia **28** (5): 1131. 2014.

53 Cross N, Melo JP, Feng L, Goldman JM. An optimized multiplex polymerase chain reaction (PCR) for detection of BCR-ABL fusion gene mRNAs in hematologic disorders. Leukemia **8** (1): 186–9. 1994.

54 Lee W-I, Kantarjian H, Glassman A, Talpaz M, Lee M-S. Quantitative measurement of BCR/abl transcripts using real-time polymerase chain reaction. Annals of Oncology **13** (5): 781–8. 2002.

55 Branford S. Monitoring after successful therapy for chronic myeloid leukemia. ASH Education Program Book **2012** (1): 105–110. 2012.

56 McCann S. Interview with Susan Branford on Monitoring CML (audio): June 2013 [podcast]. http://www.multiwebcast.com/_ehapodcast/medias/25810_s_branford. mp3, 2012.

57 Rai KR, Sawitsky A, Cronkite EP, Chanana AD, Levy RN, Pasternack BS. Clinical staging of chronic lymphocytic leukemia. Blood **46** (2): 219–34. 1975.

58 Binet JL, Auguier A, Dighiero G, Chastang C, Piguet H, Goasguen J. A new prognostic classification of chronic lymphocytic leukemia derived from a multivariate survival analysis. Cancer **48** (1): 198–206. 1981.

59 Chiorazzi N. Implications of new prognostic markers in chronic lymphocytic leukemia. ASH Education Program Book **2012** (1): 76–87. 2012.

60 Hallek M. Signalling the end of chronic lymphocytic leukaemia: New frontline treatment strategies. Blood **122** (23): 3723–34. 2013.

Chapter 8

'If you prick us, do we not bleed?'

Bleeding and blood clotting

Introduction*

William Shakespeare and many others recognized the connection between trauma and bleeding, and the association of bleeding with childbirth is well established. However, even though the associations are well known, understanding the mechanism of blood clotting is relatively recent. Although every medical student is familiar with modern concepts of blood clotting, and residents/fellows/trainees are fully conversant with contemporary theories, the unravelling of the complex mechanisms of blood clotting we owe to biochemists rather than to haematologists. The history of blood coagulation has already been well told (1–12), so I shall concentrate primarily on advances since 1965.

Blood clotting disorders

Antithrombin deficiency

It is almost 160 years ago that Rudolf Virchow (1821–1902) enunciated his famous triad of factors which contribute to thrombosis, namely, alterations in blood flow, changes in blood constituents, and changes in the blood vessel wall (13). Virchow's triad is still useful in determining the possible causes of thrombotic disease. Issues such as age, surgery, immobilization, pregnancy, and cancer also contribute to increased risk of thrombosis (14). Although in 1905 the German physiologist Paul Morawitz (1879–1936) proposed the concept that antithrombin (AT) (15) was responsible for the loss of thrombin activity after blood clotting, it was not until 1965 that Olave Egeberg (16) described a family with AT deficiency and a high incidence of venous thrombosis. AT is localized on the surface of endothelial cells and is stimulated by heparin. A number of mutations of AT have been described since Egeberg's initial report (14), and these mutations give rise to either functional defects in AT or reduced plasma levels of AT.

---

* William Shakespeare, *The Merchant of Venice*, Act III, Scene I.

Protein C deficiency and Protein S deficiency

The discovery of AT deficiency prompted further research and, by the mid-1970s, Protein C, a vitamin K-dependent protein with powerful anticoagulant properties in its activated form (APC) was isolated (17). Protein C was subsequently shown to be activated by thrombomodulin, which is found in high concentrations in the capillary bed. The activation of Protein C also depends on the endothelial Protein C receptor, and Protein S, an APC cofactor that was described in 1977 by Richard Di Scipio (18). Then, in 1981, a family with recurrent venous thrombosis and heterozygous Protein C deficiency was described (19), and subsequently Protein S deficiency was discovered (20). In clinical practice, however, the majority of patients with unexplained thrombosis do not have APC deficiency.

Purpura fulminans

Purpura fulminans is a devastating disease in children that results in disseminated intravascular coagulation that leads to digital necrosis (which often requires amputation), multi-organ failure, and a high mortality rate. In 1997 and 2000, Owen P. Smith and colleagues described an acquired deficiency of Protein C in children with meningococcal sepsis and purpura fulminans. Smith suggested that the outcome might be significantly improved by the administration of Protein C concentrates (21). Then in an open-label study, he and his colleagues demonstrated a reduction in mortality and fewer amputations than predicted in the group receiving Protein C concentrates (22). They also suggested that the benefits of Protein C concentrates may reflect the anticoagulant and the anti-inflammatory properties of the Protein C pathway (Figure 8.1).

Factor V Leiden

Although it had been known for a long time that there was an inherited tendency to thromboses in certain families, it was Björn Dahlbäk's observations and investigations which lead to widespread screening of individuals and families with venous thromboembolic disease (VTE). In 1993 Dahlbäk described a family with probable APC resistance (23). It was subsequently demonstrated that the defect in this and other families with VTE was due to a single G-to-A substitution in the gene for Factor V. This mutation, located at nucleotide position 1691, resulted in an amino acid change at position 506 in the protein; the mutated protein is termed 'Factor V Leiden' (24).

The discovery of Factor V Leiden and a number of other gene mutations leading to an increased tendency to VTE opened the floodgates of thrombophilia investigations (25). Subsequently, a diagnostic panel for thrombophilia testing

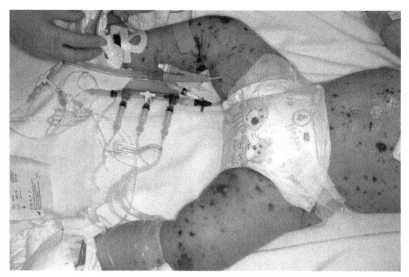

Fig. 8.1 Purpura fulminans in a baby with a widespread petechial and ecchymotic rash.

Reproduced by kind permission of Professor Owen Smith. Copyright © 2016 Owen Smith.

was proposed (26), and testing for thrombophilia became widespread during the late 1990s and early 2000s. It now appears that, with the common inherited thrombophilias mentioned in this section, the increased risk of VTE is relatively low (27). If a patient with thrombosis is diagnosed as being homozygous for deficiency in Factor V Leiden, Protein C, or Protein S, thrombophilia screening of siblings may be useful. Such screening is especially important if pregnancy is contemplated or oral contraception anticipated. The diagnosis of anti-phospholipid syndrome may lead to the institution of treatment for VTE in the case of recurrent miscarriages, but data supporting this approach is limited (28). Most agree that thrombophilia investigations should not be carried out on all patients who are heterozygous for mutations associated with VTEs.

Does Factor V Leiden provide a survival advantage?

Historically, blood loss and severe infections have been two major causes of maternal death; thus, Dahlbäk and Pelle G. Linquist have suggested that gene mutations that lower the risk of severe bleeding or infections could provide a survival advantage. Consequently, Factor V Leiden, which is present in up to 5% of Caucasian populations, may actually be a beneficial mutation, since it confers a lower risk of severe blood loss in association with delivery. In addition, Factor V Leiden carriers may have a survival advantage during sepsis.

Accordingly, Dahlbäk and Linquist suggest that the high prevalence of Factor V Leiden may be the result of one or more evolutionary selection advantages (29).

Economy class syndrome

Since air travel became popular 60 years ago and mass tourism became popular worldwide, the association between flying and VTE has become the subject of heated debate. It was thought at one stage that thrombophilia screening would be the answer and eliminate the 'economy class syndrome'. However, a detailed analysis by John T. Philbrick and colleagues of studies from 1966 to 2005 from Medline, the Cochrane Central Registry of Controlled Trials, and the Database of Abstracts of Reviews of Effects showed that there is a general risk of symptomatic VTE from prolonged air travel and that all travellers should avoid dehydration and frequently exercise leg muscles, although VTE prophylaxis is not required on a flight of less than 6 hours, provided there are no known risk factors. Travellers with one or more risk factors for VTE should wear compression stockings and consider low molecular weight heparin for flights of more than 6 hours. However, low molecular weight heparin has not been demonstrated to be effective in this setting, although its efficacy has been demonstrated elsewhere. Philbrick and colleagues favour the use of compression stockings over anticoagulants because of the risk of bleeding associated with anticoagulants and do not find aspirin of any benefit as prophylaxis against VTE in this or any other setting (30). Many airlines, on the other hand, favour the use of prophylactic aspirin, as it is available orally, whereas low molecular weight heparin needs to be injected subcutaneously.

Heparin-induced thrombocytopenia

Heparin-induced thrombocytopenia (HIT) is a relatively common and dangerous syndrome which in a subset of patients can cause thrombosis and is associated with significant morbidity and a high mortality rate. Before the diagnosis was recognized, the paradox was that, in many patients, a thrombotic tendency was accentuated by the continuation or increasing doses of heparin. As in many areas in medicine, the diagnosis remains clinical, supported by confirmatory laboratory tests (31). The diagnostic criteria include new or worsening thrombosis, thrombocytopenia (a drop in platelet count to $<100 \times 10^9/l$ or a drop of >50% from the patient's baseline platelet count), exclusion of other causes of thrombocytopenia, and the resolution of thrombocytopenia after the cessation of heparin (31).

HIT is caused by the production of an IgG antibody against a complex formed by heparin and a cytokine called Platelet factor 4 and which binds to the platelet surface (32). Once the HIT antibody has bound to the complex, the Fc portion of the antibody can then bind to the platelet Fc receptor and thus trigger the activation and aggregation of platelets. Platelet activation leads to the production of microparticles which promote coagulation (Figure 8.2). The subsequent thrombocytopenia is largely due to clearance of activated platelets by the reticulo-endothelial system (33). The immune response and the associated arterial and venous thrombotic events are more frequent with administration of unfractionated heparin than with the administration of low molecular weight heparin.

Treatment of HIT is difficult, even if a diagnosis is made quickly. The clinical diagnostic triad should be supported by functional tests, of which heparin-induced platelet aggregation is the most common (34). Heparin should be stopped immediately, and alternative anticoagulation provided. Danaparoid in therapeutic doses or an argatroban infusion is recommended at the initial stage (35) but subsequently anticoagulation with warfarin should be maintained for

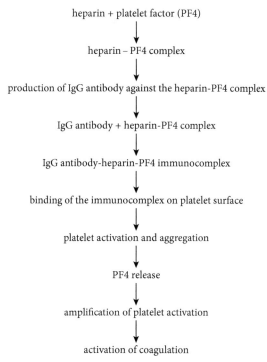

Fig. 8.2 Pathophysiology of heparin-induced thrombocytopenia.

Reproduced from Franchini M (2005). Heparin-induced thrombocytopenia: an update. *Thrombosis Journal* **3**:14, doi:10.1186/1477-9560-3-14. Reproduced under the terms of the Creative Commons Attribution License 2.0 (http://creativecommons.org/licenses/by/2.0). Copyright © 2005 Massimo Franchini.

3–6 months, as thrombotic events may occur for some time after discontinuation of heparin.

Thrombosis and cancer

Cancer is the most important disease in which patients manifest thrombotic episodes, as a sign of the underlying malignant state. Unfortunately, the discovery of inherited abnormalities of the clotting mechanism, together with the association of thrombophilia with widespread tourist travel, has thrown some doctors off the scent of an undiagnosed cancer, with possible catastrophic consequences for patients.

Von Willebrand disease

Von Willebrand disease, which is characterized by varying levels of mucocutaneous bleeding, is the most common inherited bleeding disorder. Three types of von Willebrand disease are generally recognized: type 1 is caused by a reduction in plasma levels of von Willebrand factor, type 3 is caused by a complete loss of the factor, and type 2 is caused by normal or reduced plasma levels of von Willebrand factor with defective function. However, even though the mechanisms underlying the disease may have been unravelled, diagnosis of type 1 von Willebrand disease continues to be difficult (36). As Evan Sadler said in a recent interview: 'Type 1 vWD [von Willebrand disease] is NOT a disease unless there is abnormal bleeding . . . many people who have a vWF [von Willebrand factor] level of <50 µg/dl do not bleed . . . it is important not to "over-medicalize" people with a low vWF level and who do not bleed excessively' (37) (Figure 8.3).

As type 1 von Willebrand disease accounts for 75% cases of von Willebrand disease, clearly it is important to diagnose it correctly (38). In 2005 the Scientific and Standardization Committee of the International Society on Thrombosis and Haemostasis published criteria for the diagnosis of type 1 von Willebrand disease (39), and in 2010 the same group published a questionnaire and bleeding score for the diagnosis of inherited bleeding disorders (40). However, Sadler says that, although the antigen tests for von Willebrand factor are very good, the functional assays (generally assessed as cofactor activity with ristocetin, an antibody that causes platelet agglutination only in the presence of functional von Willebrand factor) are not easily standardized and remain poor (39). Another variable is the fact that low levels of von Willebrand factor are seen in people with Group O blood (41). It has been suggested that this phenomenon is due to an increased rate of clearance of von Willebrand factor in people with this blood type (42).

The von Willebrand factor is a large multimeric glycoprotein stored in Weibel–Palade bodies in endothelial cells and in megakaryocytes. It promotes

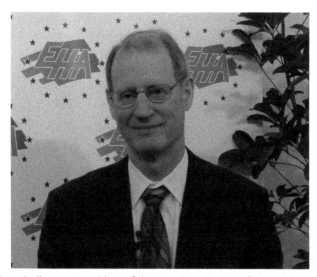

Fig. 8.3 Evan Sadler, past president of the American Society of Hematology.

Reproduced by kind permission of the European Haematology Association (EHA) and Dr E. Sadler.

platelet adhesion and aggregation and controls the half-life of Factor VIII in plasma by protecting Factor VIII from degradation. After von Willebrand factor multimers are secreted into the blood, they attach to exposed vascular subendothelium and, under shear stress, elongate into substantial strings, to which platelets adhere as part of the haemostatic process. The strings are subsequently cleaved by the metalloprotease ADAMTS13.

Type 2 von Willebrand disease, in which the function of the von Willebrand factor is defective, can be divided into four subtypes. In type 2A, the von Willebrand factor is unable to make multimers correctly or, alternatively, the multimers show increased susceptibility to cleavage by ADAMTS13, so the activity of the factor is reduced. In type 2B, there is a gain-of-function mutation in the factor, resulting in platelet binding, thrombocytopenia, and an increased rate of clearance of the factor from the plasma. In type 2M, the factor is unable to bind to platelets to activate them and, in type 2N, the factor is unable to bind to Factor VIII efficiently.

As in many areas in medicine, in spite of excellent laboratory investigations and understanding of the underlying defect, the diagnosis of von Willebrand disease remains a clinical challenge and in the end depends on a thorough history, including a family history and an over-the-counter drug history (aspirin is widely used and often not considered a drug), augmented by a von Willebrand factor antigen assay (37). Menorrhagia may be a presenting feature of von

Willebrand disease type 1; however, it can be difficult to obtain clear-cut diagnostic criteria for menorrhagia. Menstrual bleeding in excess of 80 ml per month is considered excessive; however, subjective determination of menstrual blood loss can be inaccurate. Thus, while menorrhagia is more prevalent in women with von Willebrand disease than in women without the disease, it does not seem worthwhile perform a screen for von Willebrand disease on all women who present with menorrhagia. As Sadler says: 'Empirical treatment (such as oral contraception or the Mirena coil) of menorrhagia is probably just as good in women with type 1 vWD as in the normal population' (38).

According to David Lillicrap's review, little has changed in terms of the treatment of von Willebrand disease in the last 20 years. Desmopressin will provide haemostatic coverage for minimally invasive surgery, and tranexamic acid is also effective. All patients in whom desmopressin is contemplated should have a test, followed by measurement of levels of the von Willebrand factor antigen, von Willebrand factor activity, and Factor VIII, prior to surgery (43). Concentrates of von Willebrand factor are available and appear safe and effective. If the level of Factor VIII is very low, then Factor VIII concentrates should also be given. Recombinant von Willebrand factor in combination with recombinant Factor VIII appears to provide excellent haemostatic control and is safe. Thus, although the diagnosis and management of type 1 von Willebrand factor continues to pose clinical problems, the new recombinant concentrates may herald the way forward.

Thrombotic thrombocytopenic purpura

The hereditary form of thrombotic thrombocytopenic purpura (TTP) was first described in 1960 (44). It is a rare but devastating condition characterized by thrombocytopenia, microangiopathic anaemia, fluctuating renal impairment, and fever (45). The reported incidence is six cases per million per year (46); however, there is a large overlap between haemolytic uremic syndrome (HUS) and TTP. The pathological description common to both is thrombotic microangiopathy (TMA). Cases of HUS in children are usually associated with *Escherichia coli* 0157:H7 infection. Cases in adults may be a presenting feature of systemic lupus erythematosus or occur late in pregnancy or post-partum. In some instances, calcineurin inhibitors may cause dose-dependent renal TMA (47).

Cases of so-called TTP following allogeneic stem cell transplantation do not respond to the standard therapy and should be called HSCT(for haematopoietic stem cell transplantation)-associated TMA; the majority of these cases are secondary to infection. Recently, Sonata Joedele and colleagues demonstrated that proteinuria and elevated markers of complement activation were associated with a poor outcome in patients with HSCT-associated

TMA; this finding suggests that early and prolonged intervention in such cases might be beneficial (48).

Plasma exchange and plasma infusion have been used since the 1960s for the treatment of TTP, since it was thought that something was either missing or present in the plasma of affected patients. Then, in 1998 a deficiency of the metalloprotease ADAMTS13 was reported and believed to be the necessary criterion for the diagnosis (49, 50). A lack of ADAMST13 is believed to result in a persistence of large von Willebrand factor multimers, which are the most biologically active forms of the factor, resulting in increased thromboses. Over time, however, it appeared that a deficiency of ADAMS 13 was not present in all patients who otherwise fulfilled the criteria for the diagnosis of TTP. Thus, the diagnosis of TTP remains a clinical one although, somewhat surprisingly, James George in his article entitled 'How I treat patients with thrombotic thrombocytopenic purpura: 2010' does not mention a blood film as a clinical diagnostic tool. In addition, he maintains that all plasma products are equally effective and that the decision to proceed with plasma exchange should be made before ADAMTS13 levels are obtained, although patients with high levels of ADAMT13 autoantibodies may have a poor prognosis. Response to treatment is defined as a rise in the platelet count. High-dose corticosteroids are indicated in the absence of infection, and rituximab (anti-CD20) has been used effectively when infection is present.

Although there is much excellent investigative work on ADAMTS13, a deficiency of ADAMTS13 is not universal among patients with TTP nor does it necessarily identify which patients will respond to plasma exchange. As George points out: 'Much about TTP has changed in the past 10 years, but much more needs to be achieved' (47). He also says, somewhat controversially, that there is no evidence that platelet transfusions are detrimental, although we have always tended not to give platelets when a diagnosis of TTP was suspected.

Platelet function abnormalities

Platelet function abnormalities were first described by Eduard Glanzmann (1887–1959) in the early twentieth century and, although rare, have led to significant understanding of platelet physiology and pathology. These disorders can be congenital or acquired, and the clinical history, physical examination, and evaluation of a well-made blood film and full blood count should still be in the forefront of the evaluation of patients suspected of having such a defect. Physical examination to rule out any systemic disease, as well as inspection of mucosal surfaces for the detection of bleeding, should be carried out.

From a clinical point of view, platelet function defects can be classified as mild or severe (51). The requirement of a blood transfusion, as intervention to stop bleeding, or for anaemia caused by excessive bleeding, all point towards the possible diagnosis of a platelet function abnormality. Two extensive reviews, one by Paula H. B. Bolton-Maggs and colleagues (51), and the other by Paquita and Alan T. Nurden (52), provide details of the biochemical and genetic lesions associated with platelet disorders. Deficiencies of glycoprotein mediators of platelet adhesion (Bernard–Soulier syndrome) and aggregation (Glanzmann's thrombasthenia), related to the glycoprotein Ib-IX-V complex and the integrin alpha 2b beta 3, respectively, have been well studied. Affected gene chromosomal locations include Chromosomes 21, 22, 7, and 1, and some platelet function disorders, like Wiskott–Aldrich syndrome, are X-linked.

The review by Nurden and Nurden supplies a full account of the syndromes, affected gene chromosomal locations, inheritance, and phenotypes (52). Some platelet function defects may be associated with an obvious phenotype; for example, Hermansky–Pudlak syndrome is associated with albinism, because both the defect in delta (dense) granules in the platelets and the absence of skin, hair, and iris pigmentation are due to abnormalities of lysosomal-related organelles. Mutations in *GATA1*, which encodes a transcription factor involved in cell growth, have been associated with X-linked thrombocytopenia. Abnormalities in *MPL*, which encodes the thrombopoietin receptor, may result in thrombocytopenia and aplasia, and activating mutations of *MPL* give rise to familial thrombocytopenia (53). Mutations, in *RUNX1*, which encodes a haematopoietic transcription factor, are more sinister; as well as being associated with familial thrombocytopenia, affected patients have a propensity to develop acute myeloid leukaemia (54). Mutations in *GP1BA*, which encodes glycoprotein Ib, give rise to platelet-type von Willebrand disease; this form of the disease which may be difficult to distinguish from type 2B von Willebrand disease, which is due to mutations within exon 28 of the gene encoding von Willebrand factor. Thrombocytopenia is usually mild in platelet-type von Willebrand disease, and bleeding is due to rapid clearance of von Willebrand factor multimers from the blood.

Therapies for blood clotting disorders

Anticoagulants

Aspirin

Willow bark was probably used in Mesopotamia (modern-day Iraq), as documented by the 'Middle Egyptians' in the Ebers Papyrus. The Ebers Papyrus, purchased by George Ebers, who was a German Egyptologist, is a copy of a more ancient manuscript that was probably influenced by Sumerian medical practice from around 3000 BC (55). A facsimile of the Ebers Papyrus is now in Leiden University (Figure 8.4). The willow is one of many plants containing salicylates, perhaps because salicylates act as a deterrent to insect predators or help to fight contagion by inducing apoptosis of leaves.

As we have seen, serendipity has played a role in many scientific discoveries. This is also the case with aspirin and the unfolding of its mechanism of action after World War II (56). Initially, this investigation was led by the English pharmacologist Sir John Robert Vane, who won the Nobel Prize for Physiology

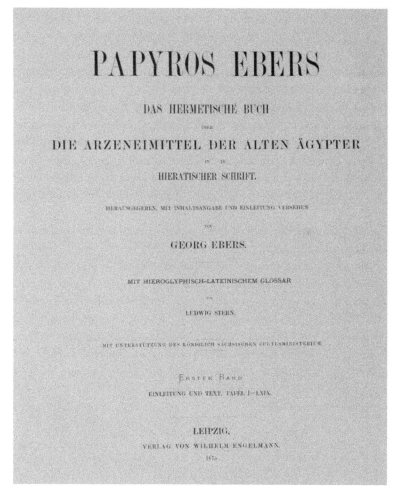

Fig. 8.4 A photograph of a facsimile of the Ebers Papyrus.

or Medicine in 1982 with Sune K. Bergström and Bengt I. Samuelsson for 'their discoveries concerning prostaglandins and related biologically active substances' (56). It was originally used for its antipyretic and analgesic properties, and many physicians who are not haematologists believe that aspirin reduces platelet numbers in peripheral blood; however, we now know that this belief is incorrect. Instead, aspirin inhibits platelet aggregation/adhesion by inactivating cyclooxygenase 1 and 2, the inactivation of which in turn halts the synthesis of thromboxane.

Aspirin is widely used in the prevention of myocardial infarction (56) and ischaemic stroke (57) and has also been shown, in both short- and long-term use, to reduce the incidence and metastatic potential of colon cancer (58, 59) (Figure 8.5). The demonstration that aspirin was effective in reducing myocardial infarction depended, to a large extent, on meta-analysis, performed by Sir Richard Peto and colleagues, of randomized clinical trials. (Meta-analysis is a statistical method whereby the results of numerous clinical trials may be analysed in order to investigate the possibility of a trend which individual trials may not observe.) Peto, the enfant terrible of epidemiology, was an unusual figure within the conservative medical profession, with long, blond hair, an open-necked shirt, and a strong sense of irony, which probably did not enhance his case with regulatory authorities when trying to establish the role of aspirin in the prevention of myocardial infarction (60, 61).

The mechanism of action of aspirin in colon cancer is unclear but may be related to activating mutations of phosphoinositide kinase, which regulates the expression of cyclooxygenase-2. As we saw in Chapter 7, imatinib, a tyrosine kinase inhibitor which changed the lives of many patients with chronic myeloid leukaemia, was almost 'lost' as a therapeutic agent. A similar fate nearly befell aspirin, when Heinrich Dreser, the CEO of Bayer, discounted the experiments of the chemist Felix Hoffman. In 1897 Ernst Eichengrün, the chief pharmacist at Bayer and who had directed Hoffman to develop aspirin, fought against Dreser to have the drug developed. In spite of this contribution, Eichengrün was subsequently written out of history, perhaps because he had fought Dreser or because he was Jewish.

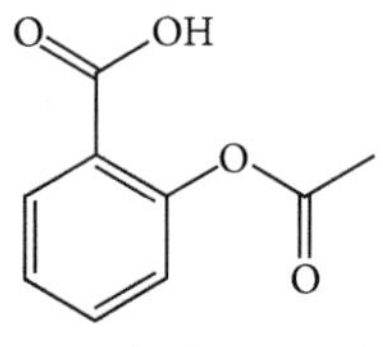

Fig. 8.5 The structural formula for acetylsalicylic acid (aspirin).

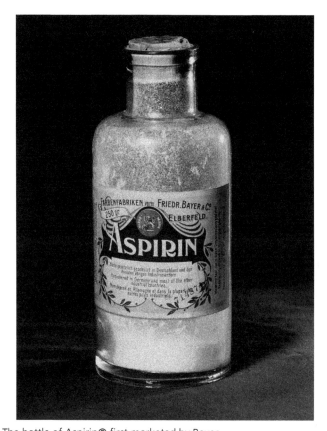

Fig. 8.6 The bottle of Aspirin® first marketed by Bayer.

Reproduced by kind permission of Bayer Healthcare AG. Copyright © 2016 Bayer Healthcare AG.

It may seem strange to us now but Bayer was originally a German company which manufactured aniline dyes. The original patent for aspirin was granted to Bayer in the United States, the United Kingdom, and throughout the British Empire. Aspirin® went on to become the biggest selling drug in the world, and many similar compounds are available today (Figure 8.6).

Warfarin

For many years we have used the vitamin K antagonist warfarin as an oral anti-coagulant to prevent or treat thromboses (Figure 8.7). In a short article, Munir Pirmohamed provides the historical context for the discovery/development of warfarin (62). It started in the 1920s, when cattle in North America and Canada developed a fatal bleeding disorder. The cattle had been eating silage made from sweet clover which contained *Melilotus alba* and *M. officinalis*. However, it took

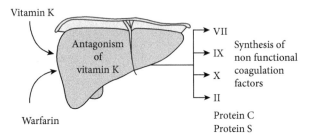

Fig. 8.7 Action of warfarin.

another 20 years before the offending substance in these plants was identified as the anticoagulant dicoumarol (63); the discovery of this compound led to the development of warfarin, which is a synthetic derivative of dicoumarol.

Warfarin is metabolized in the liver, and there are a number of polymorphisms which may alter the patient's sensitivity to a given dose of the drug. Polymorphisms of *CYP2C9* and *VKORC1* are well documented (64) as influencing the patient's response to warfarin. However, polymorphisms only account for slightly more than half of the bleeding problems associated with warfarin (65), and most patients do not have careful genetic evaluation before beginning anticoagulation.

In addition, in spite of its widespread use and low cost, there are a number of problems associated with warfarin. Patients on warfarin require frequent blood tests for monitoring, and the dose may need to be adjusted frequently, although published experience suggests that warfarin clinics run by pharmacists or nurses might be effective and less costly than those run by doctors (66–68). Warfarin also interacts with many other medications (69). Lastly, but very importantly, patient overdose is difficult to treat, and every year a number of deaths due to intracranial bleeding are reported (Figure 8.8). There is also the risk of patient non-compliance and subsequent thrombosis.

The new anticoagulants

The so-called new anticoagulants target either thrombin itself or Factor Xa, which cleaves the thrombin precursor to make thrombin (70). Thus, they either inhibit thrombin activity or the generation of thrombin. Three new anticoagulants are currently licensed: rivaroxaban and apixaban are Factor Xa inhibitors, and dabigatran is a thrombin prodrug, that is, it requires metabolic activation to become a thrombin inhibitor. Unlike warfarin, these drugs are not metabolized

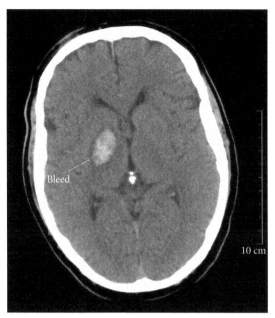

Fig. 8.8 A brain CT showing an intracranial haemorrhage in a patient taking warfarin.

Reproduced from McCann S, Foà R, Smith O, and Conneally E., *Haematology: Clinical Cases Uncovered*, Second Edition, Wiley/Blackwell, Oxford, UK, Copyright © 2009, with permission from John Wiley and Sons Ltd.

in the liver but instead must be excreted by the kidneys; dabigatran has the greatest potential for overaccumulation, as 80% of the drug is cleared in this way. On the positive side, these new anticoagulants have fewer drug interactions than warfarin does and thus can be given at a fixed dose without monitoring.

But are these new anticoagulants as good as the tried and tested warfarin? In short, they are. In atrial fibrillation, all three have been shown to be as good as warfarin, and safer, with fewer intracranial bleeds. However, dabigatran and rivaroxaban are associated with more gastrointestinal bleeding than warfarin is. In their review, Jeffrey Weitz and Peter Gross deem the advent of the new anticoagulants to be a 'giant step forward' but also say that not all patients need to change from a stable and well-managed warfarin schedule (70). As more physicians and patients become familiar with the new anticoagulants, the role of these drugs in the continuing attempts to prevent thrombotic diseases will no doubt increase. Nonetheless, a recent article in *Drugs and Therapeutics Bulletin* made the bizarre statement that patients should make an informed choice as to which anticoagulant to choose. How it could be thought that a patient could possibly make an informed choice when experienced physicians still have difficulty making such a decision is baffling (71).

Platelet transfusions

For young physicians in Western countries, platelet transfusions on demand have become normal practice, and we certainly could not have embarked on the treatment of haematological malignancies or seen the success of stem cell transplantation without them. This development is, however, fairly recent, and there are still some unresolved issues regarding the use of platelet transfusions. The fact that there have been more than 20 papers/recommendations for platelet transfusions in the last 10 years perhaps reflects the lack of consensus among clinicians concerning this procedure.

Transfusions of platelets on demand did not become widely available until the mid-1960s. Valentina Gazzaniga and Laura Ottini provide a good historical account of the discovery and description of platelets and agree that Giulio Bizzozzero (1846–1901) was the first to clearly establish the nature of platelets (72). Platelets can be collected from single donor by apheresis, or a number of units can be pooled. Platelet concentrates can be made by the platelet-rich plasma method or the buffy coat method, with no difference in efficacy when stored for up to 7 days. Universal leukodepletion may reduce the incidence of platelet refractoriness due to alloimmunization. Platelets collected by apheresis may also reduce the risk of alloimmunization by reducing the exposure to multiple donors.

Prophylaxis versus therapeutic platelet transfusions

The debate about platelet transfusions as prophylaxis or therapy rages, fast and furious. The death of a patient from bleeding secondary to thrombocytopenia because of inadequate platelet support is a tragedy for both the patient and the doctor. Guidelines may be useful when deciding on a policy to be instituted in a department but should not be used in place of clinical experience. Sherrill Slichter, for example, writing in 2007, suggested that the use of a platelet count of $10 \times 10^9/l$ as a transfusion trigger both is haemostatically efficacious and is cost-effective in reducing platelet transfusion requirements; however, she also stated that platelet counts higher than that could be required in specific situations, for example, a platelet count of $50–100 \times 10^9/l$ for patients undergoing surgery or major trauma, and a count of $100 \times 10^9/l$ for neurosurgical procedures (73). She reinforces her point in an editorial in the *New England Journal of Medicine*, stating that there are fewer intracranial bleeds if prophylactic platelet transfusions are given than when they are not used. She also pointed out in the editorial that data published in medical journals are usually the result of carefully conducted studies in academic centres and may not reflect the 'real world' (74). A careful history may not always be possible in a critically ill patient, and the ingestion by a patient of frequently used drugs which interfere with platelet function, such as aspirin, may mean that a platelet count of greater than $10 \times 10^9/l$ is required for haemostasis. Moreover, although the automated platelet count was another important development in haematology (75), it is important to stress that haematologists still need to examine a well-made blood film, as platelet clumping can provide spurious low platelet counts.

Platelet transfusions in critically ill patients

Recently, Lani Lieberman and colleagues have addressed the issue of platelet transfusions in critically ill patients (76). They suggested that prophylactic platelet transfusions may be indicated in patients with platelet counts between $10 \times 10^9/l$ and $20 \times 10^9/l$, basing their conclusions on data from chemotherapy-induced thrombocytopenia (77, 78). However, as there is little data on this subject from intensive care units, the authors suggested that a randomized controlled clinical trial should be conducted. However, it is difficult to envisage how such a trial could be performed in an ethical manner.

Thrombolytic therapy for myocardial infarction and cerebrovascular accidents

In the last 15–20 years, thrombolytic therapy has become a major discussion point in the acute treatment of myocardial infarction and cerebrovascular accidents. Comparisons are made with placebo or primary percutaneous coronary intervention (PCI; coronary angioplasty), and thrombolysis for acute myocardial infarction. The choice of intervention depends on an accurate diagnosis, requiring urgent access to intracranial imaging in the case of a cerebrovascular accident to rule out bleeding, and whether cardiac surgery is available on site. In the case of ischaemic stroke, it seems that the administration of intravenous tissue plasminogen activator, recombinant or not, results in an improved patient outcome if given up to 4.5 hours after the event (79). Two large studies in 2002 and 2003 indicate that PCI is superior to thrombolytic therapy for the treatment of acute myocardial infarction (80, 81). Primary PCI has now become the treatment of choice for an acute myocardial infarct if performed in a hospital, with or without surgery onsite. Thrombolysis is now only administered in the Western world if the time to reach a primary PCI centre exceeds 2 hours, in which case it is administered and the patient is then transferred to a primary PCI centre for immediate intervention if they do not appear to have reperfused, or for coronary angiography the next day if they have reperfused.

Conclusion

Bleeding and clotting are major causes of mortality and morbidity: even beyond inherited clotting disorders and the recent upsurge in economy class syndrome, cerebrovascular accidents and myocardial infarction are two of the main causes of death worldwide. In spite of advances in our understanding of the mechanisms of haemostasis and thrombosis in health and disease, we still have much to learn and a lot more to do to reduce the incidence of bleeding and clotting.

References

1 Greaves M. Coagulation history, Oxford 1951–1953. British Journal of Haematology 107 (1): 22–32. 1999.

2 Melanby J. The coagulation of blood. Journal of Physiology 38 (1): 28–112. 1908.

3 Howell WH. Theories of blood coagulation. Physiology Reviews 15 (3): 435–70. 1935.

4 Owren PA. The Coagulation of Blood: Investigations of a New Clotting Factor. Gunderson, Oslo, 1947.

5 Biggs R and Macfarlane RG. Human Blood Coagulation and its Disorders. Blackwell Scientific Publications, Oxford, 1953.

6 Douglas AS. Anticoagulant Therapy. Blackwell Scientific Publications, Oxford, 1962.

7 Quick AJ. Haemorrhagic Diseases and Thrombosis. Second edition, Kempton, London, 1966.

8 Tullis JL. Clot. Thomas, Springfield, IL, 1976.

9 Macfarlane RG. Human Blood Coagulation, Haemostasis and Thrombosis. Second edition. Blackwell Scientific Publications, Oxford, 1976.

10 Wintrobe MM. Blood, Pure and Eloquent. McGraw-Hill Inc., New York, NY, 1980.

11 Ratnoff OD. Disorders of Hemostasis. Saunders, Philadelphia, PA, 1996.

12 Forbes CD. The Early History of Haemophilia. Chapman & Hall Medical, London, 1997.

13 Virchow RLK. Phlogose und Thrombose im Gefäßsystem. Gesammelte Abhandlung zur Wissenchartlichen Medzin. Staatsdruckerei, Frankfurt, 1865.

14 Dahlbäk B. Advances in understanding pathogenic mechanisms of thrombophilic disorders. Blood 112(1): 19–27. 2008.

15 Morawitz P. Die Chemie der Blutgerinnung. Ergebnisse der Physiologie 4 (1): 307–422. 1905.

16 Egeberg O. Inherited antithrombin deficiency causing thrombophilia. Thrombosis et Diathesis Hemorrhagica 13: 516–30. 1965.

17 Stenflo JA. A new vitamin K-dependent protein: purification from bovine plasma and preliminary characterization. Journal of Biological Chemistry: 251; 355–363. 1976.

18 Di Scipio RG, Hermodson MA, Yates SG, Davie EW. A comparison of human prothrombin, factor IX (Christmas factor), factor X (Stuart factor), and protein S. Biochemistry: 16 (4): 698–706. 1977.

19 Griffin JH, Evatt B, Zimmerman TS, Kleiss AJ, Wideman C. Deficiency of protein C in congenital thrombotic disease. Journal of Clinical Investigation 68 (5): 1370–3. 1981.

20 Comp PC, Esmon CT. Recurrent venous thromboembolism in patients with a partial deficiency of protein S. New England Journal of Medicine 311 (24): 1525–8. 1984.

21 Smith OP, White B, Vaughan D, Rafferty M, Claffey L, Lyons B, et al. Use of protein C concentrates, heparin and haemofiltration in meningococcus-induced purpura fulminans. Lancet 350 (9091): 1590–5. 1997.

22 White B, Livingstone W, Murphy C, Hodgson A, Rafferty M, Smith O, et al. An open-label study of the role of adjuvant hemostatic support with protein C replacement therapy in purpura fulminans associated meningococcemia. Blood 96(12): 3719–24. 2000.

23 Dahlbäk B, Carlsson M, Svensson PJ. Familial thrombophilia due to a previously unrecognised mechanism characterized by poor anticoagulant response to activated protein C: prediction of a cofactor to activated protein C. Proceedings of the National Academy of Sciences of the United States of America 90(3): 1004–8. 1993.

24 Bertina RM, Koeleman BP, Koster T, de Ronde H, van der Velden PA, Reitsma PH. Mutations in blood coagulation factor V associated with resistance to activated protein C. Nature 369 (6475): 64–7. 1994.

25 Poort SR, Rosendaal FR, Reitsma PH, Bertina RM. A common genetic variation in the 3'-untranslated region of the prothrombin gene is associated with elevated plasma prothrombin levels and an increase in venous thrombosis. Blood 88 (10): 3698–703. 1996.

26 Reitsma PH, Rosendaal FR. Past and future of genetic research in thrombosis. Journal of Thrombosis and Haemostasis 5 (Suppl 1): 264–9. 2007.

27 Middeldorp S, Coppens M. Evolution of thrombophilia testing. http://www.sah.org.ar/Revista/numeros/vol17.n.extra.26.37.pdf, 2013.

28 Linquist PG, Dahlbäk B. Carriership of Factor V Leiden and evolutionary selection advantage. Current Medicinal Chemistry 15 (15): 1541–4. 2008.

29 Philbrick JT, Shumate R, Siadaty MR, Becker DM. Air travel and venous thromboembolism: A systematic review. Society of Internal Medicine 22 (1): 107–14. 2007.

30 Cines DB, Bussel JB, McMillan RB, Zehnder JL. Congenital and acquired thrombocytopenia. ASH Education Program Book 2004 (1): 390–406. 2004.

31 Franchini M. Heparin-induced thrombocytopenia: An update. Thrombosis Journal 3 (1): 14. 2005.

32 Kelton JG, Smith JW, Warkentin TE, Hayward CP, Denomme GA, Horsewood P. Immunoglobulin G from patients with heparin-induced thrombocytopenia binds to a complex of heparin and platelet factor 4. Blood 83 (11): 3232–9. 1994.

33 Chong BH. Heparin-induced thrombocytopenia. Journal of Thrombosis and Haemostasis 1 (7): 1471–8. 2003.

34 Warkentin TE. Heparin-induced thrombocytopenia: Pathogenesis and management. British Journal of Haematology 121 (4): 535–55. 2003.

35 Watson H, Davidson S, Keeling D. Guidelines for the diagnosis and management of heparin-induced thrombocytopenia. British Journal of Haematology 159 (5): 528–40. 2012.

36 Branchford BR, Di Paola J. Making a diagnosis of VWD. ASH Education Program Book 2012 (1): 161–7. 2012.

37 McCann S. Interview with Evan Sadler Is von Willebrand factor always associated with bleeding (video): January 2012 [podcast]. http://www.multiwebcast.com/_ehapodcast/medias/17900_Evan%20Sadler_master.mp3, 2012.

38 Sadler JE, Mannucci PM, Berntorp E, Bochkov N, Boulyjenkov V, Ginsburg D, et al. Impact, diagnosis and treatment of von Willebrand disease. Journal of Thrombosis and Haemostasis **84** (2): 160–74. 2000.

39 Sadler JE, Rodeghiero F. Provisional criteria for the diagnosis of vWD type1. Journal of Thrombosis and Haemostasis **3** (4): 775–7. 2005.

40 Rodeghiero F, Tosetto A, Abshire T, Arnold DM, Coller B, James P, et al. ISTH/SCC bleeding assessment tool: A standardised questionnaire and a proposal for a new bleeding score for inherited bleeding disorders. Journal of Thrombosis and Haemostasis **8** (9): 2063–5. 2010.

41 Volt AJ, Masser-Bunschaten EP, Zarakova AG, Haan E, Kruitwagen CL, Sixma JJ, et al. The half-life of infused factor VIII is shorter in haemophiliac patients with blood group O than in those with blood group A. Journal of Thrombosis and Haemostasis **83** (1): 65–9. 2000.

42 Castman G, Eikenboom JCJ. ABO blood group also influences the von Willebrand factor (VWF) antigen level in heterozygous carriers of VWF null alleles, type 2 N mutations Arg854Gln, and the missense mutation Cys2362Phe. Blood **100** (5): 1927–8. 2002.

43 Lillicrap D. von Willebrand disease: Advances in pathogenic understanding, diagnosis and therapy. ASH Education Program Book 2013 (1): 254–60. 2013.

44 Mansouri Taleghani M, von Krogh AS, Fujimura Y, George JN, Hrachovinová I, Knöbl PN, et al. Hereditary thrombotic thrombocytopenic purpura and the hereditary registry. Hämostaseologie **33** (2): 138–43. 2013.

45 Crawley JTB, Scully MA. Thrombotic Thrombocytopenic purpura: Basic pathophysiology and therapeutic strategies. ASH Education Program Book 2013 (1): 292–9. 2013.

46 Schulman I, Pierce M, Lukens A, Currimbhoy Z. Studies on thrombopoiesis. Blood **16** (1): 943–57. 1960.

47 George JN. How I treat patients with thrombotic thrombocytopenic purpura: 2010. Blood **116** (20): 4060–9. 2010.

48 Joedele S, Davies SM, Lane A, Khoury J, Dandoy C, Goebel J, et al. Diagnostic and risk criteria for HSCT-associated thrombotic microangiopathy: A study in children and young adults. Blood **124** (4): 645–53. 2014.

49 Furlan M, RoblesR, Galbusera M, Remuzzi G, Kyrle PA, Brenner B. et al. Von Willebrand factor-cleaving protease in thrombotic thrombocytopenic purpura and the haemolytic uremic syndrome. New England Journal of Medicine **399** (22): 1578–84. 1998.

50 Tsai HM, Lian ECY. Antibodies to von-Willebrand factor-cleaving protease in acute thrombotic thrombocytopenic purpura. New England Journal of Medicine **339** (22): 1585–94. 1998.

51 Bolton-Maggs PHB, Chalmers EA, Collins PW, Harrison P, Kitchen S, Liesner RJ, et al. A review of inherited platelet disorders with guidelines for their management on behalf of UKHCDO. British Journal of Haematology **135** (5): 603–33. 2006.

52 Nurden P, Nurden AT. Congenital disorders associated with platelet dysfunctions. Journal of Thrombosis and Haemostasis **99** (2): 253–63. 2008.

53 Ding J, Komatsu H, Wakita A, Kato-Uranishi M, Ito M, Satoh A, et al. Familial essential thrombocythemia associated with a dominant-positive activating mutation of the c-MPL gene which encodes for the receptor for thrombopoietin. Blood **103** (11): 4198–200. 2000.

54 Geddis AE, Kaushansky K. Inherited thrombocytopenias: Toward a molecular understanding of disorders of platelet production. Current Opinion in Pediatrics **16** (1): 15–22. 2004.

55 Jeffreys D. Aspirin: The Remarkable Story of a Wonder Drug. Bloomsbury, London, 2005.

56 Rothwell PM, Price JF, Fowkes FGR, Zanchetti A, Roncaglioni MC, Tognoni G, et al. Short-term effects of daily aspirin on cancer incidence, mortality and non-vascular death: Analysis of the time course of risks and benefits in 51 randomised trials. Lancet **379** (9826): 1602–12. 2012.

57 Baigent C, Blackwell L, Collins R, Emberson J, Godwin J, Peto R, et al. Aspirin in the primary and secondary prevention of vascular disease: Collaborative meta-analysis of individual participant data from randomised trials. Lancet **373** (9678): 1849–60. 2009.

58 Kaur J, Sanyal SN. PI3Kinase/Wnt association mediates COX2/PEG (2) pathway to inhibit apoptosis in early stages of colon carcinogenesis: Chemoprevention by diclofenac. Tumor Biology **31** (6): 623–31. 2010.

59 Chan AT. COX-2 expression in adenoma: An imperfect marker for chemoprevention. Gut **59** (5): 568–9. 2010.

60 Chen ZM, Sandercock P, Pan HC, Counsell C, Collins R, Liu L, et al. Indications for early aspirin use in acute ischemia stroke: Analysis of 40,000 randomized patients from the Chinese Acute Stroke Trial and the International Stroke Trial. Stroke **31** (6): 1240–9. 2000.

61 News Analysis. A-rise, Sir Richard (p>0.001). Tobacco Control **8** (3): 242.

62 Pirmohamed M. Warfarin: Almost 60 years old and still causing problems. British Journal of Clinical Pharmacology **62** (5): 509–11. 2006.

63 Stahmann MA, Huebner CF, Link KP. Studies on the hemorrhagic sweet clover disease. V. Identification and synthesis of the hemorrhagic agent. Journal of Biological Chemistry **138** (2): 513–27. 1941.

64 Kamal F, Khan TI, King BP, Frearson R, Kesteven P, Wood P, et al. Contribution of age, body size and CYP2C9 genotype to anticoagulant responses to warfarin. Clinical Pharmacology and Therapeutics **75** (3): 204–12. 2004.

65 Sconce EA, Khan TI, Wynne HA, Avery P, Monkhouse L, King BP, et al. The impact of CYP2C9 and VKORC1 genetic polymorphisms and patient characteristics upon warfarin dose requirements: Proposal for a new dosing regimen. Blood **105** (7): 2329–33. 2005.

66 Ellis RF, Stephens MA, Sharp GB. Evaluation of a pharmacy-managed warfarin-monitoring service to coordinate inpatient and outpatient therapy. American Journal of Hospital Pharmacy **49** (2): 387–94. 1992.

67 Foss MT, Schoch PH, Sintek CD. Efficient operation of a high-volume anticoagulant clinic. American Journal of Health System Pharmacy **56** (5): 443–9. 1999.

68 Burns N. Evaluation of warfarin dosing by pharmacists for elderly medical in-patients. Pharmacy World Science **26** (4): 232–7. 2004.

69 Pirmohamed M, James S, Meakin S, Green C, Scott AK, Walley TJ, et al. Adverse drug reactions as a cause of admission to hospital: Prospective analysis of 18,820 patients. British Medical Journal **329**: 258–64. 2006.

70 Weitz JI, Gross PL. New oral anticoagulants: Which one should my patient use? ASH Education Program Book 2012 (1): 536–40. 2012.

71 **Drugs and Therapeutics Bulletin**. Apixaban and rivaroxaban for stroke prevention in AF. Drugs and Therapeutics Bulletin **52** (1): 6–9. 2014.

72 **Gazzaniga V, Ottini L.**The discovery of platelets and their function. Vesalius **7** (1): 22–6. 2001.

73 **Slichter SJ**. Evidence-based platelet transfusion guidelines. ASH Education Program Book 2007 (1): 172–8. 2007.

74 **Slichter SJ**. Eliminate prophylactic platelet transfusions? New England Journal of Medicine **368** (19): 1837–8. 2013.

75 **McCann S**. Interview with David Nathan on Views of the winner of the Wallace H. Coulter Award for Lifetime Achievement in Hematology Changes I have seen in hematology practice (audio): January 2012 [podcast]. http://www.multiwebcast.com/_ehapodcast/medias/17912_David_Nathan_audio.mp3, 2012.

76 **Lieberman L, Bercovitz R, Scholapur NS, Heddle NM, Stanworth SJ, Arnold DM, et al**. Platelet transfusions for critically ill patients with thrombocytopenia. Blood **123** (8): 1146–52. 2014.

77 **Stanworth SJ, Estcourt LJ, Powter G, Kahan BC, Dyer C, Choo L, et al**. A no-prophylaxis platelet-transfusion strategy for hematologic cancers. New England Journal of Medicine **368** (19): 1771–80. 2013.

78 **Estcourt L, Stanworth S, Doree S, Hopewell S, Murphy MF, Tinmouth A, et al**. Prophylactic platelet transfusions for prevention of bleeding in patients with haematological disorders after chemotherapy and stem cell transplantation. Cochrane Database Systematic Review **5**: CD004269. 2012.

79 **Hacke W, Kaste M, Bluhmki E, Brozman M, Dávalos A, Guidetti D, et al**. Thrombolysis with alteplase 3 to 4.5 hours after acute ischaemic stroke. New England Journal of Medicine **359** (13): 1317–29. 2008.

80 **Aversano T, Aversano LT, Passamani E, Knatterud GL, Terrin ML, Williams DO, et al**. Thrombolytic therapy vs primary percutaneous coronary intervention for myocardial infarction in patients presenting to hospitals without cardiac surgery. Journal of the American Medical Association **287** (2): 1943–51. 2002.

81 **Keeley EC, Boura JA, Grimes CL**. Primary angioplasty versus intravenous thrombolysic therapy for acute myocardial infarction: A quantitative review of 23 randomised trials. Lancet **361** (9351): 13–20. 2003.

Chapter 9

Molecules, genes, and gene therapy

Nothing exists except atoms and empty space;
everything else is opinion.

Attributed to Democritus (*c.*460–*c.*371 BC)

Introduction

Leucippus of Miletus (*c.*460–*c.*370 BC) and Democritus (*c.*460–*c.*371 BC) are credited with the first philosophical description of the atom. Both were known to Aristotle and Plato, who apparently disliked them. Greek 'atomic theory' claimed that all matter was composed of atoms, that there was a void between the atoms, and that they were completely solid. The Greeks were very near the truth; however, it was only in 1803 AD that John Dalton put the atom on a sound scientific footing.

In the last 10–15 years, the explosion of molecular medicine has provided fresh insight into disease mechanisms. However, in spite of this revolution, the cure for many common cancers continues to elude us. Gene therapy is still not a reality for most diseases, although Arthur Nienhuis from the NIH spoke about the possible use of gene therapy for haematological diseases at an annual meeting of the American Society of Hematology in the mid-1970s. At that time it seemed very plausible, and the impression was given that gene therapy would be a reality within the next 10 years. Nienhuis reminds us, somewhat defensively but nonetheless accurately, in a review published in 2008 that it also took a long time for chemotherapy to be refined and used in daily practice (1). The culmination of the Human Genome Project in 2001 once again held the promise of great advances in medicine but, as Sir Gordon Duff said at the time: 'We have the alphabet; we now need the language' (2) (note that, although there are only 26 letters in the English language, they form over one million words). Many 'single-gene' diseases still elude our attempts at cure, and most common diseases involve many genes which interact in a complex fashion.

How did it all begin?

The publication in 1953 by James Watson and Francis Crick of the double-helix model of DNA was one of the most important discoveries of the twentieth century (3) (Figure 9.1). Now diseases could be analysed at a molecular level, the pathogenesis understood, and hopefully cures could be developed. Watson recounts that, when the paper was sent to the journal *Nature*, it was published within a very short time (4), as there was no peer review in those days. However, as with most 'discoveries', it was built on the work of many people (5). Although Watson, Maurice Wilkins, and Crick shared the Nobel Prize for Medicine or Physiology in 1962 for the discovery of the double helix, the role of Rosalind Franklin in the 'discovery' is always hotly debated.

Dublin and DNA

Watson spoke twice in Dublin in 2013; once he addressed the Royal Irish Academy and a few days later he spoke at a seminar in the biochemistry department in Trinity College, Dublin (Figure 9.2). At that time, he recalled how he had been greatly influenced by Erwin Schrödinger's book, *What is Life?* (6) (see

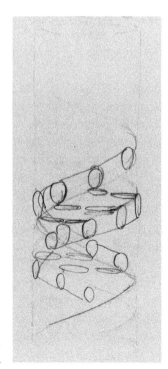

Fig. 9.1 Sketch of a DNA double helix, by Francis Crick.

Reproduced from Wellcome Library, London. Image ID: B0004367. Pencil drawing, 1953, Francis Harry Compton Crick. Library reference no.: Archives and Manuscripts PP/CRI/H/1/16. Copyright © 2015 Wellcome Library, London, UK.

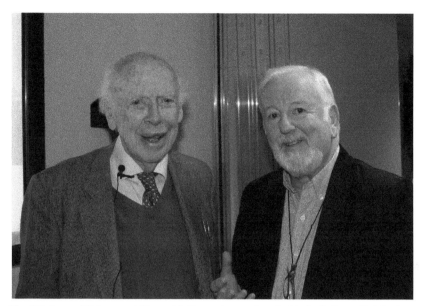

Fig. 9.2 James Watson and Shaun McCann at a seminar in Trinity College, Dublin, in 2013.

Figures 9.3 and 9.4). Many others, including Crick and Wilkins had also been inspired by Schrödinger's ideas.

Remarkably, it turns out that, in 1940, Schrödinger had been invited to Ireland by Éamon de Valera, Taoiseach (Prime Minister of Ireland) and a mathematician, to establish the Dublin Institute for Advanced Studies, and his famous book was based on lectures delivered at Trinity College, Dublin, in February 1943 (Figure 9.5). As Paul Davies, the English physicist says: 'in [this] little [book] Erwin Schrödinger set down, clearly and concisely, most of the great conceptual issues that confront scientists who would attempt to unravel the mysteries of life' (6).

In addition, the unravelling of genetics and its application to haematology owes a debt to bacteriologists such as William Hayes, a Dublin man and graduate of Trinity College, Dublin (7), who with many others elucidated the genetic events that underpin cell development and division.

Sickle cell disease: 'The first molecular disease'

The story of sickle cell anaemia (Figures 9.6 and 9.7) is well told by C. Lockard Conley in Maxwell Wintrobe's book *Blood, Pure and Eloquent* (8), where he

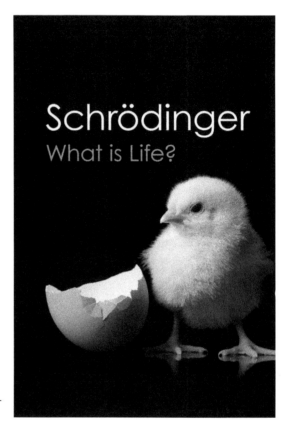

Fig. 9.3 The cover of the book *What is Life?*, by Erwin Schrödinger, Cambridge University Press © 2012.

Reproduced by kind permission of Cambridge University Press. Copyright © 2012 Cambridge University Press, UK.

refers to it as 'the first molecular disease'. From the work of Linus Pauling, Max Perutz, Vernon Ingram, and many others we now know that this devastating disease is caused by a genetic mutation which results in the substitution of a single amino acid (glutamic acid for valine) in the sixth position of the beta globin protein, and that this mutation alters the solubility of deoxygenated haemoglobin. The disease was first reported by James Herrick in 1910 (9) and since then numerous physicians and scientists have studied abnormal haemoglobins.

Although the disease occurs mainly in black Africans and Afro-Americans, the unravelling of the molecular lesion took place in the United States and the United Kingdom. Wintrobe claims this is because American physicians were accustomed to using microscopes, whereas in other countries microscopy tended to be a discipline confined to pathologists. He claims that the occurrence of the gene in the United States 'could be accounted for by the influx of blacks from Africa', carefully avoiding the word 'slavery' (8).

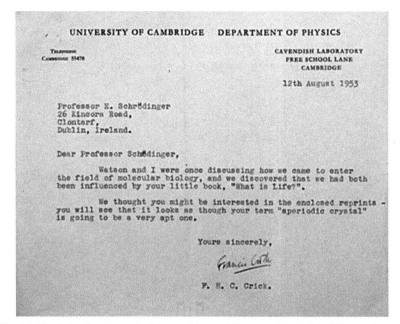

Fig. 9.4 The letter from Francis Crick and James Watson to Erwin Schrödinger, dated 12 August 1953.

Reproduced by kind permission of The Dublin Institute for Advanced Studies (DIAS). Copyright © 2016 Dublin Institute for Advanced Studies, Dublin, Republic of Ireland.

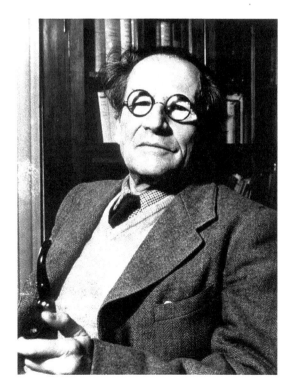

Fig. 9.5 A photograph of Erwin Schrödinger.

Reproduced with kind permission from The Dublin Institute for Advanced Studies (DIAS). Copyright © 2016 Dublin Institute for Advanced Studies, Dublin, Republic of Ireland.

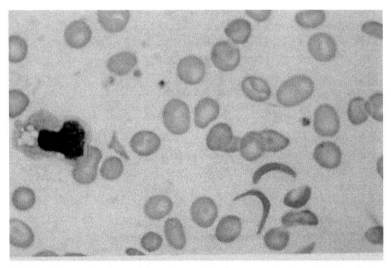

Fig. 9.6 A photograph of a peripheral blood film from a patient with sickle cell disease, showing sickled red cells.

Reproduced from McCann S, Foà R, Smith O, and Conneally E., *Haematology: Clinical Cases Uncovered*, Second Edition, Wiley/Blackwell, Oxford, UK, Copyright © 2009, with permission from John Wiley and Sons Ltd.

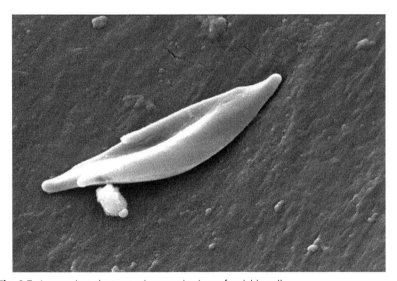

Fig. 9.7 A scanning electron microscopic view of a sickle cell.

Reproduced from Centers for Disease Control and Prevention, Public Health Image Library (PHIL), Image ID#11687, CDC/Sickle Cell Foundation of Georgia: Jackie George, Beverly Sinclair, 2009, available from http://phil.cdc.gov/phil/details_linked.asp?pid=11687

However, in spite of the thorough biochemical and molecular elucidation of the genetic mutation in sickle cell disease, severe morbidity and premature death remain associated with this disease. In 1994 Orah Platt and colleagues published a paper in the *New England Journal of Medicine*, reporting that the median survival for males with sickle cell disease was 42 years and was 48 years for females (10). They also found that the probability of premature death increased dramatically over the age of 20 years. Causes of death included sepsis and haemorrhagic stroke; in addition, rather disconcertingly, sudden and unexpected death occurred in 45 patients and, in the majority of these cases, death occurred during the course of a painful episode with or without 'chest syndrome'. In the United Kingdom, where they are rightly proud of the National Health Service, the life expectancy of individuals with sickle cell disease is still about 55 years. The only positive prognostic indicator seems to be elevated levels of fetal haemoglobin in adults, as these have been shown to be associated with improved long-term survival.

New understandings of the pathophysiology of sickle cell disease

Until recently, the pathophysiology of sickle cell disease was believed to result from sickle haemoglobin polymerizing under hypoxic conditions and thus causing the occlusion of blood vessels. However, in 2006 A. Kyle Mack and Gregory J. Kato reported that haemoglobin released during haemolysis mopped up nitric oxide, thus increasing vasoconstriction and inhibiting blood flow (11). Nitric oxide is synthesized by endothelial cells. It causes vasodilation, increases regional blood flow, and suppresses platelet aggregation, the expression of cell adhesion molecules, and the secretion of procoagulant proteins. Endothelial cells may also be dysfunctional in sickle cell disease, so that there is reduced production of nitric oxide. Further evidence of chronic endothelial damage comes from the circulation of microparticles derived from endothelial cells (12). The production of reactive oxygen species in patients with sickle cell disease results in membrane damage and mitochondrial dysfunction. Repeated oxidative stress induces an inflammatory response, causing further cellular injury (13). All of these phenomena contribute to the clinical problems experienced by patients with sickle cell disease.

New problems in sickle cell disease

Although people with sickle cell disease do not have a normal life expectancy, it is evident that survival has improved in the last 50 years. Improved survival has led to new problems, however, such as alloimmunization to red cell antigens, and iron overload. Red cell transfusion remains the cornerstone of treatment for sickle cell disease, and the vast majority (>90%) of adults with sickle cell disease have received at least one blood transfusion. An active blood transfusion programme has been shown to prevent many of the clinical problems associated with sickle cell disease, such as stroke and acute chest syndrome (13). However, alloimmunization remains a major issue in patients with sickle cell disease. It is multifactorial, and determinants include the genetic heterogeneity of the Rh blood group system, especially in people of African descent. However, now high-throughput platforms can detect blood group antigens such as Rh, Kell, and Duffy, among others. In a 2013 review, Stella Chou predicts that the use of molecular technologies for patients and donors will reduce the rate of alloimmunization in sickle cell disease patients (14). Such use is a good example of how new molecular techniques can improve the quality of clinical care for patients.

As mentioned, another problem associated with an increased life expectancy in sickle cell disease is iron overload from repeated blood transfusions. However, the issue of iron overload is significantly different in sickle cell disease, compared with that in thalassaemia major. Firstly, in the latter disease, most of the haemolysis takes place within the bone marrow (ineffective erythropoiesis), whereas in sickle cell disease most of the haemolysis is intravascular. Secondly, in thalassaemia major, the level of hepcidin (a polypeptide hormone that is synthesized in the liver and which reduces uptake of dietary iron and reduces exit of iron from macrophages) is reduced, thus leading to an increase in iron absorption from the gastrointestinal tract; but this is not the case in sickle cell disease. Nonetheless, iron overload continues to be a major contributor to premature death in sickle cell disease (15). Most problems relate to liver iron, with little cardiac or endocrine involvement. Serum ferritin measurements have been traditionally used to assess iron overload in sickle cell disease but such measurements can be confusing, as ferritin is an acute phase reactant. Although MRI is the 'gold standard' for assessing iron overload, it is an expensive technique and not available in many countries where sickle cell disease is prevalent. Iron overload can be treated or prevented by chelation therapy. Unfortunately, data from large prospective randomized trials are lacking. Compliance is another issue and, although iron chelators mobilize iron from the liver and other organs, the end point of trials should be the impact of iron chelation on life expectancy (15) rather than the ability to increase iron excretion.

Pulmonary hypertension in sickle cell disease

Although pulmonary hypertension was first described at autopsy in 1891 (16), it has only been recognized relatively recently as a major clinical problem and may be present in 6%–11% of patients with sickle cell disease (17). It is now clear that pulmonary hypertension reduces life expectancy in patients with sickle cell disease (18). Unfortunately, there have been no randomized controlled clinical trials to evaluate intervention in sickle cell disease patients with pulmonary hypertension; so, at present, the approach is to manage the patient aggressively with blood transfusion and perhaps hydroxyurea. Limiting the number of painful crises may help to reduce or contain pulmonary hypertension.

New treatments for sickle cell disease

Drugs to alter the clinical profile of sickle cell disease are now in common use. Hydroxyurea (hydroxycarbamide) has been known since the late nineteenth century but only received a licence for use in sickle cell disease in adults from the FDA in 1998 (19). It raises the level of fetal haemoglobin and reduces the amount of sickle haemoglobin in the erythrocytes of patients, thus ameliorating symptoms. Its precise method of action is disputed but it undoubtedly improves patients' quality of life (20) and may increase life expectancy (21). A study reported in *Blood* in 2004 claimed that hydroxyurea is well tolerated in children for at least 8 years (22). However, because it is a chemotherapeutic agent, its use in children should be carefully monitored for long- term toxicity. The drug Siklos (hydroxycarbamide) has been licensed by the European Medicines Agency for the treatment of sickle cell disease, in children over the age of 2 years, in adolescents, and in adults. The European Commission granted marketing authorization throughout the European Union for Siklos on 29 June 2007. Other agents which are aimed at pathophysiological abnormalities in sickle cell disease include anti-inflammatory agents, nitric oxide, arginine, and drugs which inhibit cell adhesion. Although numerous clinical trials are being conducted, none of these approaches have yet been widely adopted (13).

Haematopoietic stem cell transplantation in sickle cell disease

The most obvious curative approach to sickle cell disease is allogeneic haematopoietic stem cell transplantation. Experience is limited because of the cost of the procedure, its toxicity, and the need for expert medical personnel. In many countries where sickle cell disease is common, medical services are not well developed and therefore haematopoietic stem cell transplantation is not an option. The problem always to be faced when haematopoietic stem cell transplantation is considered is, should it be carried out early in the course of the disease, with the attendant risks, or should the procedure be carried out later, when the patient has suffered significant toxicity from the underlying disease? The first allogeneic haematopoietic stem cell transplantation for sickle cell disease was carried out in 1984 by F. Leonard Johnson and colleagues. However, the child who underwent the transplant had acute myeloid leukaemia as well as sickle cell disease (23). Emmanuel Payen and Phillipe Leboulch reviewed the results of haematopoietic stem cell transplantation for sickle cell disease and report that, between 1996 and 2012, 300 children (most of whom were <16 years of age) received allogeneic haematopoietic stem cell transplantation, worldwide (24). The disease-free survival was between 85% and 90%. It should be remembered, however, that the donors may have be heterozygous for sickle haemoglobin and that the best outcome is seen when a state of stable mixed donor/recipient chimaerism exists following haematopoietic stem cell transplantation. The option of haematopoietic stem cell transplantation may become increasingly acceptable with improved techniques of tissue typing, the use of umbilical cord blood, and haplo-identical transplants. However an inexpensive, widely available, and effective treatment is still awaited for patients with sickle cell disease.

Political issues and sickle cell disease

Jean Raphael has pointed out that the amount of money spent on research in sickle cell disease in the United States is significantly less than that spent on cystic fibrosis (25). He explains that this difference is due to the facts that there is no 'champion' for sickle cell disease and the affected Afro-American population is largely underserved. He also says that, while providing information, motivation, and advice on behavioural skills to families of patients with sickle cell disease is extremely important, compliance problems may actually result from a fear of the possible carcinogenicity of hydroxycarbamide. This situation may also be the case in countries other than the United States. The main risk period for serious complications of sickle cell disease in the United States is the transition from adolescence to adulthood, as patients may find difficulty in finding a physician willing to provide medical care. The treatment of patients with sickle cell disease therefore still poses many problems, even in so-called developed countries.

Thalassaemia

The thalassaemias are the result of quantitative abnormalities of the proteins which contribute to the make-up of human haemoglobin. Thalassaemia is the commonest monogenetic disease in humans and should be amenable to cure with haematopoietic stem cell transplantation or gene therapy. The disorder is found in Mediterranean countries, the Middle East, the Indian subcontinent, and throughout South East Asia (Thailand, Malaysia, and southern China).

However, with current migration patterns, patients with thalassaemia can be found in any country. In the mid-1970s, David Weatherall and John Paul provided the first description of a gene deletion instigating a human disease (alpha thalassaemia), a finding arrived at independently by Yuet Wei Kan at the University of California. Kan, a geneticist, is regarded as a pioneer of applying biology and genetics to clinical medicine. Apart from his work on thalassaemia, he was the first to describe DNA polymorphism.

The physician with whom the disorder thalassaemia is associated most frequently is Sir David Weatherall. He is a clinician/scientist with a career spanning over 50 years and who provided a clearer understanding of the pathophysiology of this syndrome. Even more importantly, his work led to improvements in patient management. He also developed worldwide cooperation in the diagnosis and management of the disorder. Weatherall's earlier method of in utero detection of beta thalassaemia was refined in 1982 when he published a DNA-based method for first-trimester diagnosis. It is now widely used and has significantly reduced the incidence of the disorder in many countries; for example, in Cyprus, the number of children born with thalassaemia was almost zero by the late 1980s.

In 1989 he founded the Institute for Molecular Medicine in Oxford which, on the occasion of his retirement, was renamed the Weatherall Institute of Molecular Medicine. He was awarded the prestigious Lasker Award in 2010 and the American Society of Hematology presented him with the Wallace H. Coulter award in 2013.

Clinical interventions in thalassaemia

In thalassaemia, there is a marked increase in iron uptake, and the problems of iron overload greatly exceed those seen in sickle cell disease. Blood transfusion contributes to iron overload in both conditions. Increased iron absorption from the gastrointestinal tract appears to be secondary to low hepcidin levels, as described in 'New understandings of the pathophysiology of sickle cell disease'. Hepcidin, a small peptide hormone that degrades the iron transporter ferroportin, was discovered in the year 2000 and controls iron absorption and plasma levels of iron. Hepcidin moves iron from the interior of enterocytes and macrophages to the circulation. Two proteins produced by erythroid precursors, growth differentiating factor 15 (26) and twisted gastrulation protein (27) may mediate hepcidin production in beta thalassaemia. Irrespective of the molecular control of iron, it is important to note that iron overload in beta thalassaemia can lead to significant clinical problems even in the absence of blood transfusions.

Iron chelation is effective but compliance may be a problem. Since Weatherall demonstrated that overnight infusion was as effective as the daily infusions described by David Nathan, desferrioxamine became the recommended initial therapy. Oral deferiprone or deferasirox are widely used, and combinations of desferrioxamine and deferiprone have been used but toxicity is increased. As with sickle cell disease, we need healthcare workers who are competent in the diagnosis and care of people with thalassaemia.

Hepcidin antagonists are currently under investigation in animal models of iron overload and may be a useful therapeutic intervention in humans in the future.

Gene therapy

Most people think of gene therapy as the insertion of a normal gene for a defective one, resulting in the correction of the underlying disease. However, those involved in haematopoietic stem cell transplantation will tell you that it is the ultimate form of gene therapy. The eradication of haemopoiesis in the recipient and the infusion of haemopoietic stem cells from the donor is the essence of haematopoietic stem cell transplantation, and immune tolerance ensues. Most recipients can discontinue immunosuppressive therapy after 6 or 12 months, and the donor graft remains stable, with DNA evidence of complete donor haematopoiesis.

Gene therapy: Techniques and setbacks

In a recent review, Sanjukta Misra outlined the possible approaches for gene therapy in human diseases: insertion of a normal gene into a non-specific location, the swapping of a normal for an abnormal gene by homologous recombination, repair of a defective gene by selective reverse mutation, or regulation of a specific gene. Insertion of a gene in a non-specific location, referred to as somatic gene therapy, is most commonly used (28). Insertion of a gene usually requires a vector, which is commonly a virus. Germline gene therapy refers to introduction of genes into sperm or eggs and is banned in most countries. However, knowing the human condition, it is possible that this line of investigation may be pursued by unscrupulous scientists. The main challenges for gene therapists are making sure the vector does not induce an immune reaction in the recipient and insuring expression of the new gene for the life of the patient.

Most investigators use ex vivo methods to deliver vectors. Normal genes are cloned into the vector and mixed with defective cells extracted from the patient. The transfected cells are then re-infused into the patient, and the disease hopefully is ameliorated or cured. Vectors which have been investigated include retroviruses, adenoviruses, adeno-associated viruses (AAVs), and herpes simplex viruses. A major cause for concern is the fact that genetic material is inserted randomly and thus may lead to insertional mutagenesis or to uncontrolled cell division and cancer. Cancer remains the major target for gene therapy, but monogenic diseases such as haemophilia, thalassaemia, and sickle cell disease are currently the most likely to benefit from gene therapy.

Misra provides a good historical review of attempts at gene therapy in humans (28) but points out two unfortunate results which proved detrimental to the progress of gene therapy as a clinical tool. The first was the death of young man in 1999 from multi-organ failure following gene therapy for ornithine transcarboxylase deficiency. His death was believed to be due to an immune reaction to the adenoviral vector (29). According to Barbara Sibbald, his death led to a lawsuit, a government investigation, the delay of some clinical trials, and the establishment of a new regulatory process for gene therapy trials in the United States. In 2002 Alain Fisher and colleagues used a retroviral vector to deliver gene therapy to children with severe combined immunodeficiency (SCID X1). Although initially the trial appeared successful, the group later reported that insertional oncogenesis resulting in clonal T-cell leukaemia had occurred in four patients (30). In 2010 Stefan Stein and colleagues reported the silencing of transgene (a transgene is a gene or genetic material that has been transferred from one organism to another) expression, and myelodysplasia with Monosomy 7, as a result of insertional activation of the viral integration site *EVI1* in human cells of two patients treated with gene therapy for chronic granulomatous disease. One patient died 27 months following the gene therapy, and the other was treated with haematopoietic stem cell transplantation (31). In 2014 gene therapy was tried again for the treatment of SCID. The investigators used a modified retroviral vector and as yet have not seen the development of leukaemia, although the follow-up has been relatively short (32). Because AAVs are not integrated into stem cell DNA, the risks of insertional mutagenesis and malignancy are significantly less than with the use of retroviral vectors (33). However, caution is required and the theoretical risk of malignancy has unfortunately become a reality in some studies.

Gene therapy and haemophilia B

Haemophilia A and B are monogenic diseases and therefore potentially amenable to gene therapy. Patients who are severely affected require frequent infusions of the missing protein, that is, Factor VIII or Factor IX. The formation of antibodies, called inhibitors, to these protein concentrates makes the treatment of such patients complicated. Therefore gene therapy could be associated with antibody formation to the missing protein or to the viral vector (34). Although haemophilia B is far less common than haemophilia A, the smaller size of the gene for Factor IX (the gene for Factor IX requires 1.4 kb of coding sequence, whereas that for Factor VIII requires 4.5 kb) and the fact that Factor IX is made exclusively in the liver make haemophilia B a more attractive proposition for gene therapy (34). AAVs have been extensively investigated as vectors since they may be constructed with modified viral envelope proteins. Federico Mingozzi and colleagues demonstrated in 2003 in a mouse model of Factor IX deficiency that gene therapy was most efficient with hepatic delivery (35), and Ou Cao provided evidence of regulatory T-cells which are capable of suppressing the immune response to the transgene (36).

Gene therapy: Success in humans

In 2011 Amit Nathwani and colleagues published a report of AAV-mediated gene transfer in haemophilia B. They infused a single dose of an AAV vector expressing a codon-optimized human Factor IX transgene into a peripheral vein in six patients with severe haemophilia B (37). The vector was administered without major immunosuppressive therapy. A short course of corticosteroids controlled immune- mediated clearance of AAV-induced hepatocytes without loss of transgene expression. Nathwani stated that: 'our results in haemophilia B patents serve as an important milestone for the field of gene therapy and have implications for the treatment of inherited and acquired disorders, where the treatment options are suboptimal or non-existent' (38). A follow-up published by Nathwani and colleagues demonstrated continued synthesis of Factor IX for 3 years and a marked reduction in the requirement for replacement therapy. No significant toxicity has been reported (39).

Data on gene therapy for thalassaemia were presented by Bluebird Bio, Inc., a clinical-stage company, at the annual meeting of the European Hematology Association in June 2014. They stated that two patients with thalassaemia were treated with their LentiGlobin in an autologous CD34+ setting. Both patients became transfusion independent and had high levels of the transgene beta-T87Q globin, a mutated version of beta globin that has been engineered for anti-sickling property, which it is hoped will be able to ameliorate the symptoms of sickle cell disease. At least three centres in the United States are about to enrol or have enrolled patients in gene therapy studies for thalassaemia and sickle cell disease. Fetal haemoglobin levels are important in both sickle cell disease and thalassaemia, and since *BCL11A* may have a direct role in silencing gamma globin expression (required for fetal haemoglobin) within the beta globin locus, it is likely to be a therapeutic target (40). Nathan claimed in 2011 (41) that since, *BCL11A* controls the regulation of fetal haemoglobin synthesis, we would have a cure for sickle cell disease and thalassaemia within 10 years. However, as yet there are no clinical trials addressing this issue. There is a lot of interest in monogenic diseases and the possibilities of gene therapy, but the study of these subjects is difficult (there were 32 authors on Nathwani's haemophilia B paper) and expensive, and there are many potential hazards.

Epigenetics in haematology

Although the word epigenetics was coined before Watson and Crick unravelled the structure of DNA, there are many different interpretations of its meaning. A conference was held in 2008 hosted by the Bradbury Conference Centre and Cold Spring Harbor Laboratory in order to come to an agreement on the definition of epigenetics. The definition agreed to was as follows: an epigenetic trait is a stable heritable phenotype resulting from changes in a chromosome without alterations in the DNA sequence. From the point of view of haematologists, epigenetic phenomena have become important in haematological malignancies. The development of high-throughput DNA sequencing has facilitated the identification of numerous genes that are implicated in haematological malignancies (42). Mutations in *DNMT3A, TET2* and *EZH2* are associated with many haematological malignancies (43). The realization that epigenetic phenomena are reversible has led to interesting therapeutic interventions. We now know that genes can be enabled or inhibited by transcription factors and that histones keep DNA in a compact form. Modifications in histones can affect gene expression, and aberrant DNA methylation is important in many malignancies. Hypomethylating agents and histone deacetylase inhibitors are used in the treatment of myelodysplastic syndrome, and hypomethylating agents may be useful in multiple myeloma. Yue Wei and colleagues have demonstrated that multiple genes regulated by Toll-like receptor genes (TLRs), which play an innate role in the immune system, are upregulated in vitro in CD34+ cells from patients with myelodysplastic syndrome. They also showed increased erythroid colony formation, in vitro, in patients with low-risk myelodysplastic syndrome following TLR inhibition (44). A clinical trial is currently being conducted to evaluate the effects of TLR2 inhibition in patients with myelodysplastic syndrome. Unravelling epigenetic abnormalities in haematological malignancies may also allow 'risk stratification' and open the door for experimental therapies for patients who fail to respond to conventional treatments (45).

Chun Yew Fong and colleagues provide a comprehensive review of epigenetics in haematology but admit that 'the rational use of targeted epigenetic therapies will require a thorough understanding of the underlying mechanisms and key interactions resulting in malignant transformation driven by aberrant epigenetic regulators' (46). However, as yet, although molecular discoveries are very important and provide insights into the development of malignant change, we still do not know the cause of the majority of haematological malignancies, and many patients still succumb to their disease in spite of novel treatments based on inhibition or suppression of the genetic or epigenetic abnormalities.

Small molecules in haematology

From a haematologist's perspective, small molecules are organic compounds with a molecular weight of <900 daltons. Because of their small size, they are easily absorbed and can cross cell membranes. Following the development of high-throughput, whole genome sequencing, and gene and microRNA expression profiling, a number of small molecules have been evaluated for efficacy in the treatment of haematological malignancies. The overwhelming success of tyrosine kinase inhibitors in the treatment of chronic myeloid leukaemia undoubtedly spurred on the development of these novel agents and introduced the term 'targeted therapy' into haematology. A good example of the therapeutic use of small molecules is the 'targeting' of the tumour suppressor gene p53. This gene, discovered in 1979, is on Chromosome 17 and functions by inhibiting the proliferation of abnormal cells. It is incriminated in 50% of human malignancies through deletion or mutation (47). The gene is mutated in 10%–20% of cases of chronic lymphocytic leukaemia, 10%–12% of cases of multiple myeloma, 3%–8% of cases of acute myeloid leukaemia, and 3% of cases of acute lymphoblastic leukaemia. The mutated gene is associated with 'high-risk' disease, which is aggressive and often resistant to conventional therapies. Small molecules have been developed to modulate the wild-type p53 or restore wild-type function to the mutated gene. These drugs have been identified by screening compounds which cause cell death and by a protein-based approach that identifies drugs that affect a target protein.

Ibrutinib is another example of a small molecule used for so-called targeted therapy. It is an orally bioavailable, small molecule inhibitor of Bruton's tyrosine kinase (BTK). It binds to and irreversibly inhibits BTK activity, thereby preventing B-cell activation and signalling and thus leading to an inhibition of the growth of malignant B-cells. BTK is required for signalling by B-cell receptors and plays a key role in B-cell maturation. It is overexpressed in a number of B-cell malignancies and is licensed for treatment of chronic lymphocytic leukaemia and mantle cell lymphoma. A number of clinical trials are underway to evaluate this agent in combination with chemotherapy.

Monoclonal antibodies in haematology

Monoclonal antibodies have had a huge impact on the diagnosis and treatment of haematological malignancies and, from a therapeutic perspective, are only superseded by the use of tyrosine kinase inhibitors in chronic myeloid leukaemia. MoAbs are monospecific antibodies which bind to the same epitope. They are used for the diagnosis of haematological diseases in immunohistochemistry and flow cytometry, where they identify CD (cluster of differentiation) antigens on or in cells. The diagnostic monoclonal antibodies usually identify abnormal expression of differentiation antigens on malignant cells and allow accurate diagnosis and comparison between laboratories.

From the therapeutic perspective, the anti-CD20 monoclonal antibody rituximab is probably the best known, as it has had a huge impact on many haematological diseases. It binds to surface CD20 on B-lymphocytes and activates the immune system, causing the death of malignant cells or enhancing the effects of concomitant chemotherapy (Figure 9.8). It induces both antibody-dependent and complement-dependent cytotoxicity, as well as apoptosis, in CD20+ cells. It received approval from the FDA in 1997 for the treatment of non-Hodgkin lymphomas and from the European Commission in 2010 for the treatment of follicular lymphoma. It is now widely used in protocols for the treatment of non-Hodgkin lymphomas, where it has been extremely effective. It and other anti-CD20 monoclonal antibodies are also used in the treatment of chronic lymphocytic leukaemia in combination with chemotherapy (48). An exhaustive list of therapeutic monoclonal antibodies is beyond the scope of this book but they are used in the treatment of many haematological malignancies, including acute myeloid leukaemia and acute lymphoblastic leukaemia. In all probability, the use of monoclonal

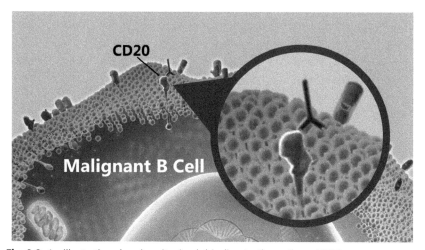

Fig. 9.8 An illustration showing rituximab binding to the antigen CD20.

antibodies will increase in haematology so that they will become part of 'conventional' treatment.

Conjugated monoclonal antibodies

Radiolabelled monoclonal antibodies (monoclonal antibodies conjugated with a radioactive particle) are agents that circulate until they find their target antigen and then deliver radioactivity to the tumour cells. Ibritumomab tiuxetan (Yttrium-90 Zevalin; Y-90 Zevalin) is probably the best-known radiolabelled monoclonal antibody (anti-CD20) and has been used in the treatment of relapsed follicular lymphoma. It was the first agent for radioimmunotherapy approved by the FDA in 2002. Y-90 Zevalin is preceded by rituximab to reduce the level of circulating malignant B-cells. As yttrium is a pure beta emitter, the danger to staff and visitors is minimal. However, there is a possibility of second malignancies such as myelodysplastic syndrome in treated patients. Brentuximab vedotin (Adcetris; anti-CD30), which is made up of an antibody attached to a chemotherapeutic agent, is showing great promise in the treatment of resistant Hodgkin disease and anaplastic large-cell lymphoma. A number of other monoclonal antibodies conjugated with chemotherapeutic agents or radioactive particles are being developed for use in haematological cancers.

Chimaeric antigen receptors in haematology

The elimination of tumour cells—the 'cure' for cancer—probably requires immune-mediated phenomena. This fact provides the basis for stem cell transplantation and for tumour vaccines. In the last few years, a number of reports have suggested that adoptive transfer of T-cells engineered to express a chimaeric antigen receptor (CAR) may be a potent therapy for otherwise refractory leukaemias (49). Although CAR-modified T-cells were first described in 1989, it is only recently that they have been successfully used to treat leukaemias (50).

Via various gene transfer technologies, autologous T-cells are engineered to express CARs. Irrespective of the gene transfer technology used, the engineered T-cells are expanded in vitro using antibodies or antigen presenting cells to engage CD3 and activate T-cells. CAR-modified T-cells recognize and bind to specific antigens. The CARs then link activated T-cells to tumour cells expressing the target antigen, and a cytotoxic T-cell response is generated.

To date, the most successful target has been CD19, as it is expressed on cells in chronic lymphocytic leukaemia and acute lymphoblastic leukaemia, and on many cells in non-Hodgkin lymphoma. Other antigens will undoubtedly be used in the future. Impressive results have been obtained in chronic lymphocytic leukaemia and B-cell acute lymphoblastic leukaemia. Continued B-cell aplasia may be a problem, however. CAR therapy may be useful in treating relapsed acute lymphoblastic leukaemia and may obviate the need for allogeneic stem cell transplantation. B-cell aplasia may be ameliorated by immunoglobulin infusions but other toxicities include cytokine release syndrome and encephalopathy. This type of treatment depends on highly trained investigators/laboratory staff and will require standardization before widespread application is possible.

Microarrays in haematology

The human diploid nucleus contains 6 billion base pairs of DNA. However, echoing the words of Sir Gordon Duff, Stefan Bohlander claims that 'we are still very far from understanding the function of the majority of this sequence (the human genome)' (51). More than 98% of our genome does not code for proteins. Because our genomes are polymorphic, we should remember this when we try to identify changes found in tumour cells. Single nucleotide polymorphisms (SNPs) are frequent but most occur in non-coding regions. However, both coding and non-coding SNPs can alter protein function.

The traditional way to examine the human genome is by chromosomal analysis, enhanced in the 1970s with banding techniques (52). Further advances were made with fluorescence in situ hybridization and comparative genomic hybridization in the 1990s (53), and mRNA or gene expression profiling, a technique developed from Southern blotting, was first described in 1982. It has subsequently been used in haematology to examine the level of expression of genes in malignant cells compared to normal cells. There are many uses for microarrays, including SNP detection (54).

DNA sequencing is the method with the highest resolution, and next-generation sequencing (a term disliked by many (55)), introduced in 2005 (56, 57), allows the exploration of large genomic regions or entire human genomes for mutations. However, although large amounts of data can be generated, the process of extraction of useful information from sequences is still a major challenge (58). Complete exome sequencing is now a commonly used technique in cancer genetics. The exome is the part of the genome formed by exons, and mutations in the exon may have a large effect on human disease. However, sophisticated software and very careful interpretation of results are required.

An example of the importance of genetic and molecular typing of haematological malignancies is provided by the classification of acute myeloid leukaemia subtype. The European Leukaemia Net groups acute myeloid leukaemia into four subdivisions based on molecular and cytogenetic data, remembering that many patients will have acute myeloid leukaemia with 'normal' cytogenetics but abnormal molecular profiles. These data may help to choose both the initial therapy and the appropriate treatment if relapse occurs (58). Another example is the classification of non-Hodgkin lymphoma subtypes. As Sandeep Dave points out, however, in spite of the explosion in molecular data which sheds light on the cell of origin in non-Hodgkin lymphoma, the correct diagnosis and prognosis for a patient with non-Hodgkin lymphoma remains a daunting clinical challenge (59). In addition, in spite of all the molecular data, we still do not know the aetiology of the vast majority of human malignant haematological diseases, although the last 10–15 years has unveiled a lot of information about the pathogenesis of these diseases. Dave, in his review, concludes that 'while in the short term, the application of genomics has complicated our understanding of lymphomas . . . In the long term . . . the genomic profile might be used to guide therapy' (59).

   Gina Zini claims that these new technologies grew out of artificial intelligence. She suggests that microarrays, gene sequencing, and protein structure predictions are only possible using computer modelling (60). She predicts that, with the use of gene profiling, the traditional diagnostic pathways will move from clinical to molecular-based diagnostic systems which may surpass clinicians in reaching a diagnosis. Mars van't Veer and Torsten Haferlach have even suggested that clinical haematologists should give up their microscopes (61), a proposition with which I do not agree (62).

Nanoparticles and nanomedicine

Nanoparticles are ultra-small particles between 1 and 100 nm in size (Figure 9.9). For comparison purposes, the size of most common proteins (e.g. albumin) and immunoglobulin molecules is also around 8–20 nm. Nanoparticles are the object of intense scientific investigation and may be relevant to drug delivery and cancer treatment. Although they seem to many of us like 'new medicine', nanoparticles have been used for thousands of years. As far back as the ninth century AD, they were used in Mesopotamia to glaze pots. In the Middle Ages and during the Renaissance they were used to create the 'lustre' effect (63).

Nanoparticles and haematology

Nanoparticles have not found their way into anti-leukaemia therapy but a publication in 2014 (64) has suggested that nanoparticles might be an effective way to deliver chemotherapy while avoiding toxicity, as the drug could be delivered directly to malignant cells. The authors claim that receptor-mediated uptake of anticancer drugs could function as an efficient drug delivery system for leukaemia treatment. They speculate that nanoparticle drug delivery could serve as a

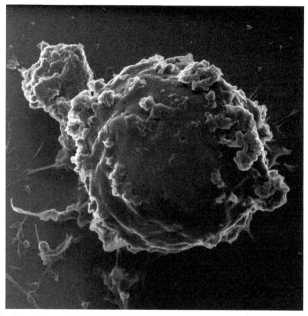

Fig. 9.9 A helium-ion microphotograph of a cell from the U266 myeloma cell line; the surface of the cell membrane has been coated with super-paramagnetic iron oxide nanoparticles.

Reproduced by kind permission of Laura Kickham and Yuri Volkov, Trinity College Dublin. Copyright © 2015 Yuri Volkov.

personalized form of therapy for patients with leukaemia. However, as Norah Campbell and colleagues state, 'Nanotechnology is an "interstitial" technoscience, the boundaries and potentialities of which are still not determined' (65).

Induced pluripotent stem cells and haematology

The existence of induced pluripotent stem cells must surely be one of the most controversial areas in medicine today. Embryonic stem cells are of great interest because they have the ability to differentiate into many different organs/cell types and therefore could be very useful in regenerative medicine. However, the use of embryonic stem cells poses ethical problems for many investigators. However, induced pluripotent stem cells should potentially also have the dual abilities of self-renewal and differentiation into all somatic cell types. In 2006 Shinya Yamanaka at the Riken Institute in Kobe, Japan, demonstrated the conversion of adult cells into stem cells by the insertion of four genes encoding transcription factors (66). For this work, he shared the Nobel Prize for Medicine or Physiology with John B. Gurdon of Cambridge, UK, in 2012. In 2014 Masayo Takahashi, an ophthalmologist from Japan, treated a patient with age-related macular degeneration with induced pluripotent stem cells and then initiated a clinical study. For this work, she was made 'Stem Cell Person of the Year'. The technique for preparing induced pluripotent stem cells has been replicated, validated, and simplified to avoid gene transfer.

Unfortunately, the story became a little murky when Haruko Obokata and colleagues, from the Center for Developmental Biology (CDB) of the Riken Institute, published two papers in *Nature* in January 2014, claiming to demonstrate a radical and relatively easy way to produce induced pluripotent stem cells (67, 68). They claimed that they had discovered a new way to produce stem cells from adult cells by applying stress. The data, however, could not be reproduced in other laboratories. In May it transpired that a similar paper had been rejected by *Nature, Science*, and *Cell* in 2012. *Nature* subsequently retracted the article in July 2014. The Riken Institute carried out an investigation, and Obokata was subsequently found guilty of scientific misconduct. Obokata initially protested her innocence but resigned in September 2014. Tragically, a co-author, Yoshiki Sasai, a noted stem cell researcher, committed suicide the same year following a sustained campaign by the media. Some claim that a swift response by the Riken Institute might have prevented Sasai's death; others say that the proposed dismantling of the CDB would be a great loss to the world of stem cell research.

The race to find new discoveries and the granting of very large amounts of money to researchers undoubtedly puts pressure on them to obtain positive results. Peer review does not always protect against fraud, but the inability of other investigators in the area to reproduce results should always arouse suspicion.

Old drugs and serendipity

The use of immunomodulatory drugs has revolutionized the treatment of multiple myeloma (69). Immunomodulatory drugs, which are functional analogues of thalidomide, were not in fact the result of extensive molecular-based research for the treatment of multiple myeloma but instead came about as a result of the promising response to thalidomide, a drug which had been known since the late 1950s. The initial use of thalidomide as an anticancer agent was due to its putative anti-angiogenic properties. As Robert A. Kyle and S. Vincent Rajkumar recall in their review, it was a plea from the wife of a patient during a phone call to Bart Barlogie which convinced him to use thalidomide, a drug which has subsequently changed the outlook for patients with multiple myeloma (70). Thalidomide and its analogues, lenalidomide being the best known, have many interesting properties, including down-regulation of key functions of myeloma cells, and modulation of interactions between myeloma cells and their micro-environment. The precise mechanism whereby they are effective in the treatment of multiple myeloma remains unknown. Thus, the serendipitous use of an 'old' drug combined with the response of an investigator to a phone call changed the world for patients with multiple myeloma.

Some 'old' drugs have achieved a second life. Bendamustine, an alkylating agent, has been manufactured in the German Democratic Republic and then Germany since 1963 but since 2008 has a licence from the FDA for the treatment of chronic lymphocytic leukaemia and indolent non-Hodgkin lymphoma. A number of clinical trials are being carried out to investigate new ways of using this 'old' drug.

Conclusion

The twenty-first century has brought many innovations in haematology, with improved diagnostic technology which may inform treatment choices for malignant diseases, and a better understanding of the genetic and epigenetic changes underlying many diseases. Unfortunately, the aetiology of most of these diseases still eludes us, and some common diseases such as sickle cell disease await simple, inexpensive, widely available curative treatment. For reasons that are often obscure, some diseases have become fashionable and attract large research financial backing, while some do not. With the advent of better technology and understanding of disease mechanisms, hopefully most haematological malignancies will enjoy the same success as the treatment of childhood acute lymphoblastic leukaemia and chronic myeloid leukaemia.

References

1 Nienhuis AW. Development of gene therapy for blood disorders. Blood **111** (9): 4431–44. 2008.

2 Duff G. Personal communication. 2014.

3 Watson JD, Crick F. A structure for deoxyribose nucleic acid. Nature **171** (4356): 737–8. 1953.

4 Watson JD. The Double Helix. A Personal Account of the Discovery of the Structure of DNA. Phoenix, London 2010. (Originally published by Atheneum Press, 1968.)

5 Pray LA. Discovery of DNA structure and function: Watson and Crick. Nature Education **1** (1): 100. 2008.

6 Schrodinger E. What is Life? Cambridge University Press 1967. (Originally published 1944.)

7 McConnell D. Personal communication. 2014.

8 Conley CL. Sickle-cell anemia: The first molecular disease, in MM Wintrobe, ed., Blood, Pure and Eloquent. McGraw-Hill, Inc., New York, NY, 1980, pp. 319–71.

9 Herrick JB. Peculiar elongated and sickle-shaped red blood corpuscles in a case of severe anemia. Archives of Internal Medicine **6** (5): 517–21. 1910.

10 Platt OS, Brambilla DJ, Rosse WF, Milner PF, Castro O, Steinberg MH, et al. Mortality in sickle cell disease: Life expectancy and risk factors for early death. New England Journal of Medicine **330** (23): 1639–44. 1994.

11 Mack AK and Kato GJ. Sickle cell disease and nitric oxide: A paradigm shift? International Journal of Biochemistry and Cell Biology: **38** (8): 1237–43. 2006.

12 Piccin A, Murphy WG, Smith OP. Circulating microparticles: Pathophysiology and clinical implications. Blood Reviews **21** (3): 157–71. 2007.

13 Vichinsky EV. Emerging 'A' therapies in hemoglobinopathies: agonists, antagonists, antioxidants, and arginine. ASH Education Program Book **2012** (1): 271–5. 2012.

14 Chou ST. Transfusion therapy for sickle cell disease: A balancing act. ASH Education Program Book **2013** (1): 439–46. 2013.

15 Porter J, Garbowski M. Consequences and management of iron overload in sickle cell disease. ASH Education Program Book **2013** (1): 447–56. 2013.

16 Collins FS, Orringer EP. Pulmonary hypertension and cor pulmonale in the sickle hemoglobinopathies. American Journal of Medicine **73** (6): 814–21. 1982.

17 Parent F, Bachir D, Inamo J, Lionnet F, Driss F, Loko G. et al. A hemodynamic study of pulmonary hypertension in sickle cell disease. New England Journal of Medicine **351** (1): 44–53. 2011.

18 Ataga K, Klings E. Pulmonary hypertension in sickle cell disease: Diagnosis and management. ASH Education Program Book **2014** (1): 425–31. 2014.

19 Segal JB, Strouse JJ, Beach CM, Haywood C, Witkop C, Park H, et al. Hydroxyurea in the treatment of sickle cell disease. Evidence Reports/Technology Assessments 165: http://www.ncbi.nlm.nih.gov/books/NBK38499/. 2008.

20 Jones AP, Davies SC, Olujohungbe A. Hydroxyurea for sickle cell disease. Cochrane Database of Systematic Reviews **2**: CD002202. 2009.

21 McCann S. Interview with Mariane de Montalembert on Sickle Cell Disease in Children (audio): Jan 2014 [podcast]. http://www.multiwebcast.com/_ehapodcast/medias/33366_m_de_montalembert_audio.mp3, 2013.

22 Zimmerman SA, Schulz WH, Davis JS, Pickens CV, Mortier NA, Howard TA, et al. Sustained long-term hematologic efficacy of hydroxyurea at maximum tolerated doses in children with sickle cell disease. Blood **103** (6): 2039–45. 2004.

23 Johnson FL, Look AT, Gockerman J, Ruggiero MR, Dalla-Pozza L, Billings FT III. Bone-marrow transplantation in a patient with sickle-cell anemia. New England Journal of Medicine **311** (12): 780–3. 1984.

24 Payen E, Leboulch P. Advances in stem cell transplantation and gene therapy in the β-hemoglobinopathies. ASH Education Program Book **2012** (1): 276–83. 2012.

25 McCann S. Interview with Jean L Raphael on Sickle Cell Disease A political issue (audio): February 2014. http://www.multiwebcast.com/_ehapodcast/medias/48168_jl_raphael_audio.mp3, 2014.

26 Tanno T, Bhanu NV, O'Neal PA, Goh SH, Staker P, Lee YT, et al. High levels of GDF15 in thalassemia suppress expression of the iron regulatory protein hepcidin. Nature Medicine **13** (9): 1096–101. 2007.

27 Tanno T, Porayette P, Sripichai O, Noh SJ, Byrnes C, Bhupatiraju A, et al. Identifica-tion of TWSG1 as a second novel erythroid regulator of hepcidin expression in murine and human cells. Blood **114** (1): 181–6. 2009.

28 Misra S. Human gene therapy: A brief overview of the genetic revolution. Journal of the Associations of Physicians of India **61** (2): 127–33. 2013.

29 Sibbald B. Death but one unintended consequence of gene therapy. Canadian Medical Association Journal **164** (11): 1612. 2001.

30 Hacein-Bey-Abina S, Garrigue A, Wang GP, Soulier J, Lim A, Morillon E, et al. Inser-tional oncogenesis in 4 patients after retrovirus-mediated gene therapy of SCID X1. Journal of Clinical Investigation **118** (9): 3132–42. 2008.

31 Stein S, Ott MG, Schultze-Strasser S, Jauch A, Burwinkel B, Kinner A, et al. Genomic instability and myelodysplasia with monosomy 7 consequent to EVI1 activation after gene therapy for chronic granulomatous disease. Nature Medicine **16** (2): 198–204. 2010.

32 Hacein-Bey-Albina S, Pai S-Y, Gaspar H, Armant M, Berry CC, Blanche S, et al. A modified γ-retrovirus vector for X-linked severe combined deficiency. New England Journal of Medicine **371** (15): 1407–17. 2014.

33 McCann S. Interview with Katherine High on Gene therapy for Hemophilia (audio): May 2013 [podcast]. http://www.multiwebcast.com/_ehapodcast/medias/25809_k_high.mp3, 2013.

34 Scott DW and Lozier JN. Gene therapy for haemophilia: Prospects and challenges to prevent or reverse inhibitor formation. British Journal of Haematology **156** (3): 295–302. 2012.

35 Mingozzi F, Liu YI, Dobrzynski E, Kaufhold A, Liu JH, Wang Y, et al. Induction of immune tolerance to coagulation factor IX antigen by in vivo hepatic gene transfer. Journal of Clinical Investigation **111** (9): 1347–56. 2003.

36 Cao O, Hoffman BE, Moghimi B, Nayak S, Cooper M, Zhou S, et al. Impact of the underlying mutation and the route of vector administration on immune responses to factor IX in gene therapy for hemophilia B. Molecular Therapy **17** (10): 1733–42. 2009.

37 Nathwani AC, Tuddenham EGD, Rangarajan S, Rosales C, McIntosh J, Linch DC, et al. Adeno-associated virus vector–mediated gene transfer in hemophilia B. New England Journal of Medicine **365** (25): 2357–65. 2011.

38 Nathwani AC. Personal communication. 2014.

39 Nathwani AC, Reiss UM, Tuddenham EGD, Rosales C, Chowdary P, McIntosh J, et al. Long-term safety and efficacy of factor ix gene therapy in hemophilia B. New Eng-land Journal of Medicine **371** (21): 1994–2004. 2014.

40 Sankaran V. Targeted therapeutic strategies for fetal hemoglobin induction. ASH Edu-cation Program Book **2011** (1): 459–65. 2011.

41 McCann S. McCann S. Interview with David Nathan on Views of the winner of the Wallace H. Coulter Award for Lifetime Achievement in Hematology Changes I have seen in hematology practice (audio): January 2012 [podcast]. http://www.multiwebcast.com/_ehapodcast/medias/17912_David_Nathan_audio.mp3, 2012.

42 Goodell MA. Epigenetics in hematology: Introducing a collection of reviews. Blood **121** (16): 3059–60. 2013.

43 Couroneé L, Bastard C, Bernard AO. TET2 and DNM3A mutations in human t-cell lymphoma. New England Journal of Medicine **366** (1): 95–6. 2012.

44 Wei Y, Dimicoli S, Bueso-Ramos C, Chen R, Yang H, Neuberg D, et al. Toll-like receptor alterations in myelodysplastic syndrome. Leukemia **27** (9): 1832–40. 2013.

45 Goodell MA, Godley LA. Perspectives and future directions for epigenetics in hematology. Blood **121** (26): 5131–7. 2013.

46 Fong CY, Morison J, Dawson MA. Epigenetics in the hematologic malignancies. Haematologica **99** (12): 1772–83. 2014.

47 Saha MN, Qiu J, Chang H. Targeting p53 by small molecules in hematological malignancies. Journal of Hematology and Oncology **6** (1): 23. 2013.

48 Bauer K, Rancea M, Roloff V, Elter T, Hallek M, Engert A, et al. Rituximab, ofatumumab, and other monoclonal anti-CD 20 antibodies for chronic lymphocytic leukemia. Cochrane Database of Systematic Reviews **11**: CD008079. 2011.

49 Grupp SA, Kalos M, Barrett D, Aplenc R, Porter DL, Rheingold SR, et al. Chimeric antigen receptor–modified T cells for acute lymophoid leukemia. New England Journal of Medicine **368** (16): 1509–18. 2014.

50 Maude SL, Shpall E, Grupp SA. Chimeric antigen receptor T-cell therapy for ALL. ASH Education Program Book **2014** (1): 559–64. 2014.

51 Bohlander SK. ABCs of genomics. ASH Education Program Book **2013** (1): 316–23. 2013.

52 Casperson T, Farber S, Foley GE, Kudynowski J, Modest EJ, Simonsson E, et al. Chemical differentiation along metaphase chromosomes. Experimental Cell Research: **49** (1): 219–22. 1968.

53 Lichter P, Tang CJ, Call K, Hermanson G, Evans GA, Housman D, et al. High-resolution mapping of chromosome 11 by in situ hybridization with cosmid clones. Science **247** (4938): 64–9. 1990.

54 Chang TW. Binding of cells to matrixes of distinct antibodies coated on solid surfaces. Journal of Immunological Methods **65** (1–2): 217–23. 1983.

55 Luzzatto L. Personal communication. 2014.

56 Margulies M, Egholm M, Altman WE, Attiya S, Bader JS, Bemben LA, et al. Genome sequencing in microfabricated high-density picolite reactors. Nature **437** (7057): 376–80. 2005.

57 Bennett ST, Barnes C, Cox A, Davies L, Brown C. Towards the $1,000 human genome. Pharmacogenetics **6** (4): 373–82. 2005.

58 Schlenk RF, Döhner H. Genomic applications in the clinic: Use in treatment paradigm of acute myeloid leukaemia. ASH Education Program Book **2013** (1): 324–30. 2013.

59 Dave SS. Genomic stratification for the treatment of lymphomas. ASH Education Program Book **2013** (1): 331–34. 2013.

60 Zini G. Artificial intelligence in hematology. Hematology **10** (5): 393–400. 2005.

61 Vant'Veer M, Haferlach T. Should clinical hematologists put their microscopes on EBay? Haematologica: **99**; 1533–1534. 2014.

62 McCann S. Comment on: 'Should clinical hematologists put their microscopes on eBay?' Haematologica **100** (1): e40. 2015.

63 Sattler KD, ed. Handbook of Nanophysics: Nanoparticles and Quantum Dots. CRC Press, Boca Raton, FL, 2011.

64 Basha R, Sabins N, Heym K, Bowman WP, Lacko AG. Targeted nanoparticles for pediatric leukemia therapy. Frontiers in Oncology **4**: 101.

65 Campbell N, Deane C, Murphy P. Advertising nanotechnology: Imagining the invisible science. Technology and Human Values: doi: 10.1177/0162243915574867. 2015.

66 Takahashi K, Yamanaka S. Induction of pluripotent stem cells from mouse embryonic and adult fibroblast cultures by defined factors. Cell **126** (4): 663–76. 2006.

67 Obokaba H, Wakayama T, Sasai Y, Kojima K, Vacanti MP, Niwa H, et al. Stimulus-triggered fate conversion of somatic cells into pluripotency. Nature **505** (7485): 641–7. 2014.

68 Obokata H, Sasai Y, Niwa H, Kadota M, Andrabi M, Takata N, et al. Bidirectional developmental potential in reprogrammed cells with acquired pluripotency. Nature **505** (7485): 676–80. 2014.

69 Singhal S, Mehta J, Desikan R, Ayers D, Roberson P, Eddlemon P, et al. Antitumor activity of thalidomide in refractory multiple myeloma. New England Journal of Medicine **341**: 1565–71. 1999.

70 Kyle RA, Rajkumar SV. Multiple myeloma. Blood **111** (6): 2962–72. 2008.

Chapter 10

The same specialty—but different approaches!

When did haematology as a specialty begin?

During a recent conversation with Professor Luke O'Neill, Professor of Biochemistry at Trinity College, Dublin, he asked me: 'When did haematology as a specialty begins?' I replied 'It was the middle of the nineteenth century, as it required the development of the microscope and good staining techniques. It evolved differently in different countries, sometimes from internal medicine and sometimes from pathology.' In this chapter, I will outline how haematology developed as a specialty in the United States, some European countries, and India. There are many other countries in which haematology is practised, so this is not an exhaustive list; rather, it is an attempt to show how the specialty has grown from different evolutionary paths.

Haematology in France

Haematology as a specialty began in France in 1931, followed by Italy in 1935, Germany in 1937, and the Netherlands in 1953. The French Society of Hematology (the first in the world) was started in 1931 by Paul Chevalier (1884–1960), and Jean Bernard was the general secretary for almost 40 years! According to Wintrobe (1), Chevalier was an original thinker. Although he began his career as a dermatologist, he turned to basic science and haematology, and his laboratory (a hut on the grounds of Hôpital Cochin) was renowned for 'une furieuse odeur de lapin' (2). He founded the European Society of Hematology with Giovanni Di Guglielmo and Paul Lambin in 1947. In 1948 he became Professor of Hematology at the University of Paris. In 1968 Jean Bernard created a 'University Institute for Hematology' similar to 'Medical Faculties' and with the same privileges but for only one discipline. The University Institute is still very active in Hôpital Saint-Louis. Successive directors were Jean Bernard, Michel Boiron, Laurent Degos, François Sigaux, and Hervé Dombret. Haematology developed into a major discipline in France when treatment for malignancies became a real possibility with chemotherapy. Unlike in Britain and the United States, there was no opposition to the establishment of a French haematology society.

Haematology in the United States of America

In his books, Wintrobe gives us a lengthy description of the setting up of the International Society of Haematology (ISH) in 1946, the American Society of Hematology (ASH) in 1958, and his opposition to both (1, 3). He initially opposed the setting up of haematology as a separate specialty, believing it should remain under the umbrella of internal medicine. He appears to have changed his mind, however, when he was elected president of the ISH and later president of ASH in 1971! Wintrobe also gives an account of haematology in many countries, although his books tend to be rather hagiographic. Of course, national societies do not always reflect the practice of haematology and indeed there can be tension between training bodies and national societies.

The establishment of ASH was also opposed by many organizations, including the American Society of Clinical Research and the American College of Physicians, both of whom believed that their meetings were adequate fora at which to present research findings. An important factor in the success of ASH was the journal *Blood*. Founded by William Dameshek in 1946, it has stood the test of time and is now arguably the foremost haematology journal in the world. The first official ASH meeting was held in Atlantic City, New Jersey, in April 1958. More than 300 haematologists met to discuss key research and clinical issues related to blood and blood diseases. The annual meeting now hosts over 20,000 delegates, about 75% coming from the United States, and the rest from South America, Europe, and further afield.

Private practice versus specialty clinics

Haematology in the United States is often practised in private institutions, and expert medical care may still depend on one's ability to pay. Hopefully, 'Obamacare' will make sure that everybody will receive expert care irrespective of income. As pointed out in Chapter 9, the amount of money spent on research in the United States on sickle cell disease is relatively small when compared to that spent on acute myeloid leukaemia.

The treatment of chronic myeloid leukaemia has been revolutionized by the introduction of tyrosine kinase inhibitors. However, in the United States, many patients with chronic myeloid leukaemia are treated by private oncologists. Some of these doctors may have little experience in treating patients with chronic myeloid leukaemia and may have difficulty interpreting laboratory results which report on the level of *BCR–ABL1* transcripts. Laboratories differ in the techniques they use, adding to difficulties in the interpretation of results. The referral of all patients with chronic myeloid leukaemia to centres which specialize in treating haematological malignancies and which have access to standardized laboratories seems preferable to the current approach (4).

Haematology in Sweden

The Swedish Society of Hematology was founded in 1962, after Sweden's hosting of the ISH annual meeting. Jan Waldenström became the first president and was the main organizer of the ISH meeting in Stockholm.

At that time, haematology was not a recognized speciality in Sweden. Clinical haematologists worked as specialists in internal medicine, oncology, and/or paediatrics. In 1975 the National Board of Health and Welfare (Socialstyrelsen) formally made haematology a 'special competence' (behörighetsämne) within internal medicine. This designation was the first step towards making haematology a specialty in its own right. From 1992 to 2013, about 250 doctors qualified as specialists in haematology in Sweden.

In 1984 The Swedish Society of Hematology began yearly specialist examinations on a voluntary basis, and this is still the case. Thus, there is no formal examination for new specialists, even though taking the examination is highly recommended. Other specialties in Sweden operate in a similar manner (5).

Laboratory haematology has never been a formal speciality in Sweden but is a competence area within pathology. Clinical immunology, transfusion medicine, and coagulation/thrombosis, on the other hand, are specialities within laboratory medicine. The majority of haematologists train in all three areas as part of their education.

Haematology in the United Kingdom

A society representing British haematologists came rather late to the scene. British haematologists had traditionally presented papers at the Association of Clinical Pathologists, the Association of Physicians, and the Pathological Society, and an attempt to form a separate scientific platform was defeated in the Royal Society of Medicine in 1950. The formation of a national society for haematology was opposed by many in Britain (6). Nonetheless, the British Society for Haematology (BSH) was formed in 1960–61.

The Pathological Society has little interest in haematology. The BSH was also established because there was a concern among haematologists of the time that its academic excellence might get lost in the College of Pathologists, a concern that turned out, in retrospect, to be exaggerated.

The Royal Society of Medicine to this day has refused to establish a haematology section, and the BSH has become the single most important voice of the specialty in the United Kingdom. It has been very successful financially and has one of the leading journals and website, *Bloodmed*. The European Hematology Association (EHA), despite its great success, had little impact on UK matters governed by BSH and the Royal College of Pathologists.

Qualification as a haematologist in the United Kingdom today requires membership of the Royal College of Pathologists; membership is usually by examination. The qualification includes examination in laboratory and clinical haematology including knowledge of haemostasis, thrombosis, and transfusion medicine. The majority of haematologists in the United Kingdom today come from a background in clinical medicine.

Haematology in India

At an EHA/Indian Society of Haematology and Blood Transfusion (ISHBT) tutorial in Kolkata in 2014, Mammen Chandy, Director of the Tata Medical Centre in that city, mentioned the importance of Yellapragada Subba Row to haematology (7); before that time, I had known little of Yellapragada Subba Row (1895–1948). He was born in Bhimavaram, Madras, and studied medicine at the Madras Medical College. After Ghandi had called on Indians to boycott British goods, Subba Row started wearing khadi surgical dress, which annoyed M. C. Bradfield, his surgery professor. Consequently, he was awarded the lesser LMS certificate, not a full MBBS degree. Following a meeting with a visiting American doctor on a Rockefeller Scholarship, and with financial assistance from his father-in-law, Subba Row travelled to Boston in 1922 (8).

His major (unrecognized) contribution was the discovery of the function of adenosine triphosphate (commonly known as ATP) as an intracellular energy source. He joined Lederle Laboratories, where he developed a method to synthesize folic acid. This research was based on work by Lucy Wills to isolate folic acid as a protective agent against anaemia. Lucy Wills, working in India, had shown how marmite was able to correct pregnancy-related anaemia which did not respond to liver extract and suggested there was another factor (called the Wills factor) which was later identified as folic acid (9). Subba Row subsequently developed the important anticancer drug, methotrexate, with considerable input from Sidney Farber.

Subba Row's colleague, George Hitchings, who shared the Nobel Prize in Physiology or Medicine in 1988 with Sir James Black and Gertrude Elion, said: 'Some of the nucleotides isolated by Subba Row had to be rediscovered years later by other workers because Fiske, (Cyrus Fiske, his supervisor at Harvard) apparently, did not let Subba Row's contributions see the light of the day.' (8). Although most of his career was spent in the United States, he was denied tenure at Harvard and remained an alien, without a green card, throughout his life.

Today in India, there are over 25 institutions where top-quality diagnostic and therapeutic haematology is practised, taught, and researched (Figure 10.1). In a publication produced by the ISHBT for their annual meeting in 2013,

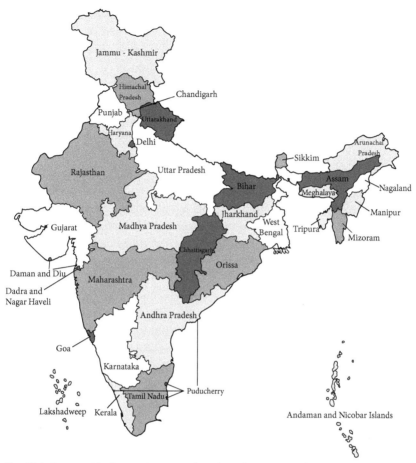

Fig. 10.1 A map of India; as Mammen Chandy said, 'When confronted with any disease, the task of providing care for such numbers is daunting.'

Reproduced by kind permission of Professor Mammen Chandy. Copyright © 2015 Mammen Chandy.

Mohan B. Agarwal gives details of 27 units/hospitals, including 16 stem cell transplant units, providing top-quality haematology services in India; he also states that the Indian Bone Marrow Transplant Registry reports data collected from 33 haematopoietic stem cell transplantation centres in India (10). The first stem cell transplant in India was carried out at the Tata Memorial Centre in Mumbai in 1983. Because haemoglobinopathies are common in India, there is a major interest in prenatal diagnosis and stem cell transplantation. The Christian Medical College in Vellore began its haematology service in the 1950s and was rehoused in 1980. Their haematopoietic stem cell transplantation pro-gramme is dedicated to patients with thalassaemia, and there is a major interest in gene therapy for haemophilia and haemoglobinopathies.

The development of haematology in India, as in many countries, depended on the vitality and interest of dedicated people. One of many examples was Betty Cowan, a Scottish physician who set up assays for vitamin B_{12} and folate in the 1960s (11). The institution in which she worked, Christian Medical College, Ludhiana, has been providing stem cell transplantation since 2007 (12). Following a meeting in Udaipur in August 2009 between the late John Goldman (1938–2013), members of the Anthony Nolan Trust, the National Marrow Donor Program, the European Blood and Bone Marrow Transplant Group, and representatives of the Indian haematopoietic stem cell transplantation community, DATRI was established to type volunteer, unrelated donors. By 2013 there were 43,000 donors on the registry and 40 unrelated haematopoietic stem cell transplantations had been performed, including 4 bone marrow harvests exported outside India (13).

India has also been at the forefront of developing generic anticancer drugs and biosimilars. Generics are drugs that are comparable to 'brand' drugs in every way except price, and biosimilars are officially approved versions of bio-pharmaceutical products made after the products' patents have expired. The Indian Council of Medical Research believes that, with 12,000 new cases of chronic myeloid leukaemia per year and a population of 1.2 billion, the number of patients on imatinib in India could reach 120,000, costing $3.2 billion annually. At present, there are at least 13 different generic forms of imatinib available at a cost of between $50 and $100 per day (12). In addition, the manufacture of generic antiretrovirals has allowed the widespread availability of HIV/AIDS treatment in developing countries. In a short report in 2010, Brenda Waning and colleagues concluded that India produced the vast majority of antiretrovirals for patients in developing countries and that the manufacture of new antiretrovirals should not be hampered by inappropriate intellectual property obligations through free-trade agreements (14). Subsequently, in 2014 the biotech company Gilead reached a landmark agreement with Medicines Patient Pool to allow the production of generic versions of Gilead's temofovir alafevamide, thus significantly reducing the cost of this drug in India, Asia, and China.

Haematology in Germany

German and French universities have had a huge influence on the Western world and especially on the USA in the nineteenth century. The so-called Prussian system encouraged the establishment of experimental laboratories in universities, arguing that these laboratories should be funded from the public purse. Although he was only head of the Prussian educational system from 1809 to 1810, Wilhelm von Humboldt was a very influential figure in German education and the development of the Prussian system. By the middle of the nineteenth century, scientists/physicians were going from the USA, Russia, and all parts of Europe to study in Germany. Many returned home and instigated educational models similar to those in Germany. The journal *Folia Haematologica* was highly respected and widely read. German professors, especially in scientific areas, were highly respected in the community.

Germany, like a number of other European countries, was greatly depleted intellectually by the emigration of Jews to America. In his biography of Oppenheimer, Monk describes three major Jewish migrations from Europe to the United States. The first took place in the seventeenth century, when Sephardic Jews emigrated from Spain and Portugal and became well established in America. The second was in the latter part of the nineteenth century, when the population of Jews in America rose from 15,000 to 280,000, most of whom were from Germany. The third migration was between 1880 and 1920, when approximately two and a half million Jews from Eastern Europe (Russia and Poland) emigrated to America (15). Finally, the Nazis forced the dismissal of many Jews from university and teaching positions and, as can be seen from the names of eminent haematologists and scientists, many emigrated to the United States because they or their spouses were Jewish. One of Germany's most important haematologists was Hans Hirschfeld, who worked at the cancer institute of the Berlin Charité. Because he was Jewish, he was forced out of his teaching position and eventually deported to the Theresienstadt concentration camp, where he died in 1944 (16). Thus, ironically, Hitler's bid to have a pure Aryan race resulted in Germany losing many of its best scientists and doctors.

Wintrobe provides the names of many eminent German haematologists in *Blood, Pure and Eloquent* (3). Unfortunately, many German physicians worked with the Nazis; in 2012 the German Medical Association formally apologized for their behaviour during and after World War II in the 'Nuremberg Declaration of the German Medical Assembly' (17).

In latter years, Germany has been associated with well-run and well-constructed clinical trials in the treatment of childhood and adult leukaemia and lymphoma. The BFM (for Berlin, Frankfurt, and Münster) study group was founded in 1975, when Hansjörg Riehm (in Berlin), Bernhard Kornhuber (in Frankfurt), and Günther Schellong (in Münster) initiated the first multicentre clinical trial. The BFM treatment concept developed by Riehm was based on a very intensive chemotherapeutic approach employing eight different drugs and led to a revolutionary increase in survival of children and adolescents with acute lymphoblastic leukaemia. Since that time, the so-called BFM treatment backbone has remained an essential component of many paediatric and adult protocols for the treatment of acute lymphoblastic leukaemia. The International BFM Study Group (I-BFM SG) was initiated in 1987. The aim was to compare treatment modalities and develop common standards for diagnosis and treatment of childhood acute lymphoblastic leukaemia. The I-BFM SG has become an important international platform for the promotion of research and clinical care for children and adolescents with leukaemia and lymphoma. In the 1920s, there were several 'Departments' and 'Laboratories' of haematology and histology, for example in the Institute of Cancer Research at the Charité, One of the first clinical 'Departments of Haematology' was established in 1961 in the 'St George Hospital' in Hamburg. Since 1976 the specialty is called 'Haematology and Medical Oncology'. Some early haematologists, such as the Königsberg pathologist Ernst Neumann, remained 'pure' scientists, but the specialty developed from the close association between scientist/pathologists, such as Rudolf Virchow, Paul Ehrlich, Artur Pappenheim, and Viktor Schilling, and many famous clinicians. Today, there is no distinction between clinical and laboratory haematology.

The German national society of haematology, the Deutsche Gesellschaft für Hämatologie, was founded in 1937. Transfusion medicine, haemostasis, and thrombosis were originally all considered part of haematology, but in 1954 the Deutsche Gesellschaft für Bluttransfusion separated from the Deutsche Gesellschaft für Hämatologie and, in 1956, the Deutsche Gesellschaft für Thrombose- und Hämostaseforschung was formed. In 1977 oncology was incorporated and the society became the Deutsche Gesellschaft für Hämatologie und Medizinische Onkologie. In the German Democratic Republic, the national society was called the Gesellschaft für Hämatologie und Bluttransfusion der DDR, a name which reflected the major interest of East German haematologists in transfusion medicine rather than in oncology. In 1990, following the reunification of Germany and the consequent dissolution of the Gesellschaft für Hämatologie und Bluttransfusion der DDR, every member of that society could apply for membership of the Deutsche Gesellschaft für Hämatologie. The first 10 years following the reunification of Germany posed many difficulties for haematologists, as West German haematologists considered themselves to be oncologists as well as haematologists, whereas the East German haematologists did not (18).

Haematology in Russia

In 2009, the hundredth anniversary of the publication of a landmark article by the pioneer Alexander A. Maximov (1874–1928) was celebrated. He worked at the Imperial Military Medical Academy in Saint Petersburg, and in 1919 he published his seminal paper 'Lymphocyte as a common stem cell for different mammalian blood cell in embryonic and post-fetal development', in which he hypothesized the existence of a common blood cell progenitor, in other words, a haemopoietic stem cell (19). This concept laid the ground for bone marrow transplantation, as well as for modern methods of cell therapy.

In 1924, this Russian-born morphologist, working in Chicago, used extensive histological findings to identify a singular type of precursor cell within mesenchyme that develops into different types of blood cells, so-called mesenchymal stem cells (20). This important observation was built upon when Andrew J. Becker, Ernest A. McCullagh, and James E. Till demonstrated the clonal nature of marrow cells in the 1960s (21). An assay for examining the clonogenic potential of multipotent marrow cells was later reported in the 1970s by Alexander J. Friedenstein and colleagues (22). The first clinical trials of mesenchymal stem cells were completed in 1995, when 15 patients were injected with cultured mesenchymal stem cells to test the safety of the treatment. Currently, a number of clinical trials are being conducted to evaluate the efficacy of mesenchymal stem cells in the treatment of graft-versus-host disease following allogeneic stem cell transplantation.

Haematology in Russia developed as an interest in the treatment of haematological malignancies but later became intimately involved with transfusion medicine. The first special haematologic clinic in Moscow was organized in the 1930s by Maxim P. Konchalovsky, who was interested in anaemias, leukaemias, and bleeding disorders. The development of a major interest in transfusion medicine was accelerated by the needs of World War II.

Thanks to Andre A. Bagdasarov of the Institute of Transfusion, and Vladimir N. Shamov, a general in the military medicine service, 50,000 doctors and nurses were trained in blood component storage, blood banking, and transfusion in 1940. During the Siege of Leningrad, large numbers of soldiers and civilians received blood transfusions.

Experimental haemopoietic stem cell research at the I. Pavlov State Medical University was started in the 1970s, when Boris V. Afanasyev, with support from Tatiana S. Istamanova and Vladimir A. Almazov, opened a laboratory for culturing haematopoietic stem cells. The main research at this laboratory was focused on the biology and growth characteristics of human blood cell progenitors in patients with various haematological disorders.

The rapid evolution of experimental and clinical haematology in the 1970s and 1980s resulted in the development of bone marrow transplantation. The first allogeneic haematopoietic stem cell transplantation in an adult patient in Russia was performed in 1974 in Moscow, and the first child received a haematopoietic stem cell transplantation in 1990 in Saint Petersburg. The first allogeneic bone marrow transplantation from an unrelated donor was also carried out by Afanasyev and co-workers in 2000. In the mid-1990s, modern protocols for treating in children and adults with leukaemia were introduced to the Saint Petersburg State Medical University (now called the First State Pavlov Medical University of Saint Petersburg).

Currently, treatment of haematological patients is concentrated in Moscow and Saint Petersburg. In Saint Petersburg, haematopoietic stem cell transplantation is carried out in the Raisa Gorbacheva Memorial Research Institute for Paediatric Oncology, Hematology and Transplantation under the direction of Afanasyev (Figure 10.2). Trainees come from internal medicine; they must produce a PhD thesis before becoming a recognized haematologist, and training is carried out in Moscow, Saint Petersburg, and Kirov.

In 1992 the National Hematological Society was initiated, with a view to optimizing research into and treatment of haematological disorders. A Russian cooperative group for the treatment of acute leukaemia was formed the same year, and subsequently registries for haematopoietic stem cell transplantation

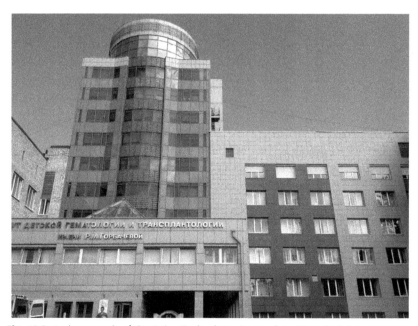

Fig. 10.2 A photograph of the Raisa Gorbacheva Research Institute in Saint Petersburg.

Reproduced by kind permission of Professor Boris V. Afanasyev. Copyright © 2015 Boris V. Afanasyev.

and for acute leukaemia were established. In 2005 and 2006, cooperative groups for aplastic anaemia and multiple myeloma were set up, and randomized trials in acute leukaemias and myelodysplastic syndromes were carried out.

In 2009 the National Society of Pediatric Hematology and Oncology was formed, again with a primary objective of developing innovative technologies for treating children with haematological disorders. The society has more than 540 members from various backgrounds, including paediatric surgery, anaesthetics, radiology, and psychology, among many others (23).

The International Society on Thrombosis and Haemostasis

Some haematologists may regret the development of separate societies to represent thrombosis/haemostasis and transfusion medicine. However, in our ever specializing world, their development was inevitable. It still behoves all haematologists to maintain a working knowledge of these areas, and there are many parts of the world where haematologists are required to deal with problems related to thrombosis/haemostasis and transfusion medicine.

In 1954, a small group of investigators used seed money from the National Heart, Lung and Blood Institute to form the International Committee on Thrombosis and Haemostasis. The committee envisioned a society that would be open to all of the researchers, clinicians, educators, and students working in the many interrelated fields of thrombosis, haemostasis, and vascular biology. In 1969 the International Society on Thrombosis and Haemostasis (ISTH) was formed. The new organizations expanded to include the emerging areas of platelet function and regulation, the mechanisms of thrombosis, fibrinolysis, and thrombolysis, and problems of thromboembolic disorders.

Today, the ISTH's impact and contributions to the understanding, prevention, diagnosis, and treatment of thrombotic and bleeding disorders span six continents. With more than 3,800 members in over 94 countries, it is now the leading thrombosis/haemostasis-related professional organization in the world.

The International Society of Blood Transfusion

Two major fields, war and infectious diseases, have provided stimuli for the development of transfusion medicine, albeit in totally different ways. Although casualties were massive in World War I, it was not until the Spanish Civil War that modern blood transfusion 'came of age'. World War II and the Korean War both had a large influence on blood collection, typing, and transfusion, so that, by the 1970s, most people took the availability of blood transfusion for granted.

Blood transfusion and its complexity came into public consciousness in the early 1980s when HIV/AIDS became an issue and especially when the disease was shown to be spread via blood and blood products. The HIV/AIDS pandemic eventually resulted in the testing of blood and blood products for antibodies to HIV, hepatitis B, and hepatitis C. In 1998 the European Agency for the Evaluation of Medicines accepted the recommendations of the Committee for Proprietary Medicinal Products for the introduction of testing of plasma pools. In 1999 the use of nucleic acid testing to detect the hepatitis C virus and HIV was introduced by many blood transfusion centres (24), although it wasn't until 2011 that nucleic acid testing for the hepatitis B virus was published (25). Meanwhile, in 2003, testing for the West Nile virus was implemented under the FDA's Investigational New Drug programme, and in 2005 the FDA approved nucleic acid testing for West Nile virus. The availability of nucleic acid testing for the virus allowed the rapid introduction of screening when an outbreak of West Nile virus, and the demonstration of its transmission through blood transfusion, became evident in 2012.

Today, emphasis is placed on the appropriate usage of blood and blood products, and the guidelines have changed dramatically since the 1980s. In many countries, training in transfusion medicine is carried out in institutions divorced from major hospitals. The use of blood transfusion for medical reasons (mostly to support combination chemotherapy) has now outstripped surgical needs, and most large hospitals have 'Transfusion Committees' which issue guidelines on blood and blood product usage and provide education to medical staff, nursing staff, and patients on the issues surrounding transfusion medicine.

The International Society for Blood Transfusion (ISBT) was founded in 1935 and, in 2009 at the annual ISBT congress, the Melbourne Declaration was made, which undertook 'to work in collaboration in international efforts to promote safe and sustainable volunteer non-remunerated blood donor programmes that foster community engagement and benefit recipients of blood and blood products'. It is to be hoped that this laudable aim will be implemented by 2020.

In 1994 the ISBT working group on automation and data processing was joined by the American Association of Blood Banks, the American Red Cross, the Department of Defence, and the Health Industry Manufacturers Association to develop a set of international standards to identify all blood and blood products. The current version of the ISBT 128 Standard Technical Specification is designed to replace the ABC Codabar and other similar Codabar-based standards with a more secure barcode which contains more information. The International Council for Commonality in Blood Banking Automation was established and given the responsibility for implementation and management of the new standard.

The ISBT is an important international organization and now has more than 1600 members. Its journal *Vox Sanguinis* is one of the most important journals in transfusion medicine and is widely read both within and outside the specialty of transfusion medicine.

The EBMT and the Center for International Blood and Marrow Transplant Research

In Europe, a group of like-minded physicians and scientists, led by Bruno Speck from Switzerland, got together in 1973 to form the EBMT. Their main focus was to encourage discussion among stem cell 'transplanters' about the clinical and scientific problems relating to stem cell transplantation and to collect and collate information from all European centres. The EBMT has been singularly successful and now has almost 500 teams from nearly 50 countries. Doctors, nurses, statisticians, and data managers meet annually and exchange clinical and research information on bone marrow transplantation. Since 2000, the EBMT has embarked on conducting clinical trials in participating countries.

On 1 July 1 2004, the Center for International Blood and Marrow Transplant Research (CIBMTR) was established. The new organization joined together the research programmes of the National Marrow Donor Program (NMDP; founded in 1986) and the International Bone Marrow Transplant Registry (founded in 1968 at the Medical College of Wisconsin). The CIBMTR collects transplant data from as many centres as possible and provides statistical analyses on a wide range of topics. There is no doubt that both the CIBMTR and the EBMT have had a major impact of the development of haematopoietic stem cell transplantation and it is difficult to believe that a worldwide transplant programme involving unrelated donors and umbilical cord blood (26) could have been successful without the international collaboration of the CIBMTR, EBMT, and NMDP.

Real improvements in the outcome of malignant haematological disorders have come about by entering large numbers of patients (leukaemia is a rare disease) in agreed protocols, knowing what disease was being treated (morphology, immunophenotyping, and genetic studies) and developments in supportive care. Not only has the outcome been improved by entering patients into randomized clinical trials, but information on drug and radiation toxicity has opened the door to treatments that are less toxic than the ones used in years past.

Haematology has developed from different backgrounds in many countries. Irrespective of its origins, haematology today is largely concerned with the understanding and treatment of malignant diseases. International cooperation and new technologies have helped to make new treatments available to patients.

Although the treatment of haematological disorders, benign and malignant, has been enhanced by international cooperative groups, appropriate treatment is still not available in many parts of the world. Hopefully, appropriate and affordable treatment for haematological diseases will become available soon.

The voice of Europe

Although the embryonic idea of a European society for haematology was evident in 1931 when Paul Chevallier created la Société Française d'Hématologie, the world's first national association dedicated to diseases of the blood, the European Association of Hematology (EHA) did not become a reality until 1991. The EHA has been important as a political body in Europe, helping to make a case for haematology as a specialty within the European Union, endeavouring to 'harmonize' haematology training in Europe, and fostering education and research.

The EHA has close ties to the European School of Haematology and the ASH and engages in education both within Europe and in many other countries through its outreach programme. However, as with other societies such as ASH and the BSH, the birth of the EHA was not without its difficulties. (For a detailed history of the formation of the EHA, see Peter Vermij's book *Fresh Blood*.) Currently the EHA holds an annual congress, and its journal is *Haematologica*.

References

1 **Wintrobe MM, ed**. Blood, Pure and Eloquent. McGraw-Hill, Inc., New York, NY, 1980.
2 **Faure CC**. Paul Chevalier. The French Pioneer of Hematology. Association Amicale des Anciens Internes en Médicine des Hôpitaux de Paris. http://www.aaihp.fr/IllustrieAncien-P-Chevalier.php
3 **Wintrobe MM**. Hematology, The Blossoming of a Science: A Story of Inspiration and Effort. Lea & Febiger, Philadelphia, PA, 1985.
4 **McCann S**. Interview with Susan Branford on Monitoring CML (audio): June 2013 [podcast]. http://www.multiwebcast.com/_ehapodcast/medias/25810_s_branford.mp3, 2012.
5 **Hast R**. Personal communication.
6 **Swan HT**. The founding of the British Society for Haematology. http://www.bloodmed.com/home/bshhistorypdf/HistoryoftheSociety1.pdf, 1989.
7 **Chandy M**. Personal communication. 2014.
8 **Bhargava BM**. Dr Yellapragada Subba Row (1895–1948): He transformed science; Changed lives. Journal of the Indian Academy of Clinical Medicine **2** (1–2): 96–100. 2001.
9 **Wills L, Bond BS**. Treatment of 'pernicious anaemia of pregnancy' and 'tropical anaemia'with special reference to yeast extract as a curative agent. British Medical Journal: **1**: 1059–64. 1931.

10 **Agarwal MB, ed**. Haematology Departments in India. Haematocon 2013. Indian Society of Haematology and Blood Transfusion. http://www.slideshare.net/ GURUINDIA2012/haematology-departmentsinindia, 2013.

11 **Wadswirth GR**. Tropical macrocytic anaemia: The investigations of Lucy Wills in India. Asia-Pacific Journal of Public Health **2** (4): 265–73. 1988.

12 **Chandy M**. A Moral Imperative: Worldwide Access to Leukaemia Treatment: John Goldman Memorial. Royal College of Physicians, London, 2014.

13 Data from DATRI. Courtesy Mr Ragu Rajagopal. DATRI 2013.

14 **Waning B, Diedrichsen E, Moon S**. A lifeline to treatment: The role of Indian generic manufacturers in supplying antiretroviral medicines to developing countries. Journal of the International AIDS Society **13**: 35. 2010.

15 **Monk R**. Inside the Centre: The Life of J. Robert Oppenheimer. Anchor Books, New York, NY, 2012.

16 **Voswinckel P**. 1937–2013. Die Geschichte der Deutschen Gesellschaft für Hämatologie und Onkologie im Spiegel ihrer Ehrenmitglieder: 'Verweigerte Ehre'. Dokumentation zu Hans Hirschfeld. DGHO, Berlin, 2012.

17 **Kolb S, Weindling P, Roelcke V, Seithe H**. Apologising for Nazi medicine: A constructive starting point. Lancet **380** (9843): 722–3. 2012.

18 **Voswinckel Peter**. Personal communication. 2014.

19 **Maximov AA**. [The lymphocyte as a stem cell common to different blood elements in embryonic development and during the post-fetal life of mammals] Folia Haematologica **8**: 125–134. 1909.

20 **Maximov AA**. Relation of blood cells to connective tissues and endothelium. Physiological Reviews **4** (4): 533–63. 1924.

21 **Becker AJ, McCulloch EA, Till JE**. Cytological demonstration of the clonal nature of spleen colonies derived from transplanted mouse marrow cells. Nature **197** (4886): 452–4. 1963.

22 **Friedenstein AJ, Chailakhyan RK, Lastinik NV, Panasyuk AF, Keiliss-Borok IV**. Stromal cells responsible for transferring the microenvironment of the hemopoietic tissues. Cloning in vitro and retransplantation in vivo. Transplantation **17** (4): 331–40. 1974.

23 **Mamev NN, Afanasyev BV**. Personal communication. 2015.

24 **Zou S, Dorsey K, Notari EP, Foster GA, Krysztof DE, Musavi F, et al**. Prevalence, incidence and residual risk of human immunodeficiency virus and hepatitis C virus infections among United States blood donors since the introduction of nucleic acid testing. Transfusion **50** (7): 1495–504. 2010.

25 **Stramer S, Wend U, Candotti D, Foster GA, Hollinger FB, Dodd RY, et al**. Nucleic acid testing to detect HBV infection in blood donors. New England Journal of Medicine **364** (3): 236–47, 2011.

26 **Ballen K, Gluckman E, Broxmeyer HE**. Umbilical cord blood transplantation: The first 25 years. Blood **122** (4): 491–8. 2013.

Chapter 11

The role of technology in haematology

Seeing is believing

17th century proverb

The microscope

Although the contribution of the ancients to our understanding of blood and the circulation was prophetic in many ways, it really was the development of the microscope which facilitated much of our present understanding. Wintrobe gives a good account of the early days of microscopy (1) but does not mention that the Romans used the so-called reading stone and that Seneca (3 BC–AD 65), the Roman playwright and Stoic philosopher, is said to have read all the books available in Rome through it. It seems that the reading stone was little more than a concave glass which magnified the image.

Zacharias Jannsen and his son Hans, in the Netherlands at the end of the sixteenth century, are credited with inventing the microscope, as they discovered that, by combining lenses in a tube, the object being scrutinized appeared to be enlarged. The invention of the microscope depended upon the skilled grinding of lenses.

Galileo Galilei (1564–1642), by working out the principles of lenses, made his first telescope in 1609, modelled after telescopes which had been produced in other parts of Europe and could magnify objects three times. His, however, could magnify objects 20 times. He was primarily interested in astronomy and physics, and it was Anton van Leeuwenhoek (1632–1723) of the Netherlands who taught himself new methods for grinding and polishing tiny lenses of great curvature so that they which gave magnifications up to 270 diameters, the finest known at that time. With his microscopes, he was the first to see and describe bacteria, yeast, and the circulation of blood corpuscles in capillaries (2). He reported his findings to the Royal Society and the French Academy although apparently his first communication to the Royal Society was greeted with mirth and derision. One member even suggested that van Leeuwenhoek was drunk when he reported his observation!

The use of more than one lens, resulting in further enlargement of the object, produced compound microscopes. Compound microscopes, however, produced chromatic and spherical aberrations. In the eighteenth century, lens makers discovered that, by combining lenses of different colour dispersions, most of the chromatic aberrations were eliminated. This observation was originally utilized in telescopes but, by the nineteenth century, chromatically corrected lenses were used in compound microscopes. English and German lens makers dominated the eighteenth century until Giovanni Battista Amici (1785–1863), an expert lens maker in Florence, Italy, produced excellent microscopes which could compete with English and German rivals. The immediate forerunner of today's microscope was monocular and had a mirror beneath the stage onto which a light was shone. A wonderful collection of such microscopes can be seen in the Galileo Museum in Florence, Italy.

A major breakthrough occurred in the middle of the nineteenth century when Ernst Abbe, working for Zeiss, formulated the Abbe sine condition, which significantly improved the optics of light microscopes. At the end of the nineteenth century, Paul Ehrlich and Dimitri Romanowsky, among others, developed staining techniques which facilitated the study of haematological conditions (see 'Staining').

Microscopes in current use are binocular and may have multiple heads for teaching. The light source is built in, and lenses have an anti-glare coating. Microprocessors are also incorporated into the microscope stand, thereby making photomicrography relatively foolproof.

The fluorescence microscope

The fluorescence microscope generates an image by using light produced by a substance, termed a fluorophore, or fluorochrome, that emits light after it has absorbed it. In fluorescence microscopy, the specimen is illuminated with light which is absorbed and then emitted at a different wavelength by the fluorophores. Most fluorescence microscopes are epifluorescence microscopes, where both excitation of the fluorophore and detection of the fluorescence are done through the objective lens. In 2014, in recognition of the scientific advances produced by the fluorescence microscope, the Nobel Prize in Chemistry was awarded to Eric Betzig, William Mourner, and Stefan Hell for the development of super-resolved fluorescence microscopy.

Immunofluorescence

Immunofluorescence uses antibodies to label a specific target antigen with a fluorescent dye such as fluorescein isothiocyanate (commonly known as FITC). Antibodies that are chemically conjugated to fluorophores are commonly used in immunofluorescence. The fluorophore allows visualization of the target distribution in the sample under a fluorescent microscope (e.g. epifluorescence and confocal microscopes).

In direct immunofluorescence, a single antibody directed against the target of interest (known as a primary antibody) is used. The antibody is directly conjugated to a fluorophore. In indirect immunofluorescence, two antibodies are used. The primary antibody is unconjugated, and a fluorophore-conjugated secondary antibody directed against the primary antibody is used to detect the unlabelled antibody. A process which addresses a number of technical issues must be adhered to if the result of the investigation is to be used diagnostically. For example, antibodies should be of high quality, and specimens should be stored in the dark.

Confocal microscopy

A technique called confocal imaging was first proposed by Paul Nipkow (1860–1940; he also invented the television) and pioneered by Marvin Minsky in 1957 (3). However, commercial production of the microscope was not feasible because the technology needed to produce useful images was not available. In 1986–87 a confocal microscope with such capabilities was built by W. Brad Amos, John G. White, and Michael Fordham in Cambridge, UK, combining laser technology, computers, and microelectronics to study images of *Caenorhabditis elegans* embryos (4).

A laser, which deflects off a mirror, is used to provide the excitation light. From there, the laser hits two other mirrors, which are mounted on motors, in order to scan the sample. Dye in the sample fluoresces, and the emitted light gets descanned by the same mirrors. The emitted light is focused onto a pinhole and is measured by a photomultiplier tube. The detector is attached to a computer which builds up the image. The image is captured onto a screen and can be stored indefinitely. A number of different software packages are available to capture the images. The sample, if needed, can be kept in the dark for years. Further advantages of the confocal microscope over previous microscopes are that single cells, cell nuclei, three-dimensional images of organisms, and binding of particles such as nanoparticles can be studied with confocal microscopy (Figure 11.1). Confocal microscopy is used predominantly for research and has not yet made its way into the diagnostic laboratory.

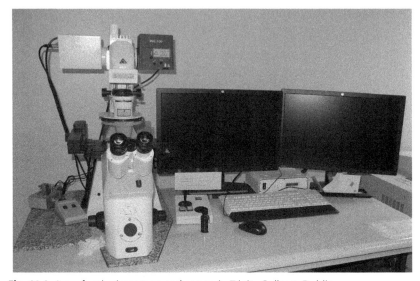

Fig. 11.1 A confocal microscope and screen in Trinity College, Dublin.

Reproduced by kind permission from Yuri Volkov and Laura Kickham. Copyright © 2015 Yuri Volkov.

Microscopy and the medical profession

The development and acceptance of microscopy in medicine was not a smooth journey. The medical profession is notoriously conservative, and their view of microscopy is a good example of such an attitude. The French public health physician Alfred Doneé (1801–78) tried very hard to interest the medical profession in microscopy. He discovered and identified *Trichomonas vaginalis* and even provided educational classes, which he financed, for doctors in Paris. However, he was largely ignored, as he was not a professor at a Paris university (5). Some even made the comment 'It is just an artefact', thinking that the use of the word 'artefact' was pejorative. However, almost everything we see microscopically is an artefact, especially if staining techniques are used. Most illness, cancer being a good example, are concepts and not what we see using a microscope. We rely on reproducible artefacts, however, to communicate accurately with each other.

Can you visualize things smaller than the wavelength of light?

Yes—although not with a light microscope. A light microscope cannot be used to distinguish objects that are smaller than half the wavelength of light. White light has an average wavelength of 0.550 μm, half of which is 0.275 μm. If two lines are closer together than 0.275 μm, they will be seen as a single line, and any object with a diameter smaller than 0.275 μm will be invisible or show up as a blur. Thus, to see tiny particles under a microscope, one must bypass light and use a different sort of 'illumination', one with a wavelength shorter than that of light. In the early 1930s, Max Knoll (1897–1969) and Ernst Ruska (1906–88) invented the electron microscope. This instrument uses electrons speeded up in a vacuum until their wavelength is extremely short, only one hundred-thousandth that of white light. Electron microscopes make it possible to view objects as small as atoms. Ernst Ruska shared the Nobel Prize for physics in 1986 with Heinrich Rohrer (1933–2013) and Gerard Binnig (1947–) for their invention of the scanning tunnelling microscope.

Although the electron microscope and the scanning electron microscope were used in haematology in the 1970s and 1980s, their use has been markedly restricted since then. At one stage, the diagnosis of hairy cell leukaemia depended on the demonstration of intracellular ribosome-lamellar complexes via the electron microscope (6), but this method has been superseded by flow cytometry.

Automated cell counting: Wallace H. Coulter

The development of automated cell counting was a major breakthrough which changed the practice of laboratory haematology. Wallace H. Coulter (1913–98) was an American electrical engineer, inventor, and businessman (Figure 11.2). He studied electronics at Georgia Tech in the early 1930s. The best known of his 85 patents is the 'Coulter principle', which provides a method for counting and sizing microscopic particles suspended in fluid. The Coulter principle states that particles pulled through an orifice, concurrent with an electric current, produce a change in impedance that is proportional to the volume of the particle traversing the orifice. This pulse in impedance originates from the displacement of electrolyte caused by the particle. Remembering his visits to hospitals, where he observed laboratory workers hunched over microscopes manually counting blood cells on haemocytometers, he concentrated on counting red blood cells. This instrument became known as the Coulter counter. This device increased the sample size 100 times more than the usual microscope method by counting in excess of 6000 cells per second. Additionally, it decreased the analysis time from 30 minutes to 15 seconds and reduced the error by a factor of approximately 10.

His invention of the Coulter counter made possible today's most common medical diagnostic test: the complete blood count, or full blood count, which

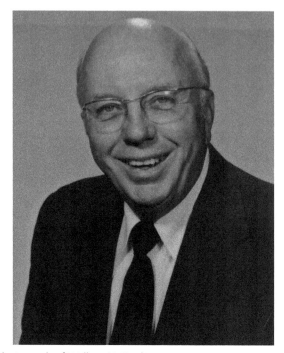

Fig. 11.2 A photograph of Wallace H. Coulter.

Image reproduced courtesy of the Wallace H. Coulter Foundation. Copyright © Wallace H. Coulter Foundation, Miami, FL, USA.

includes the red cell volume. Since the invention of the original Coulter counter, the technology has evolved to use optical and laser methods, so that accurate differential white cell counts, platelet counts, and reticulocyte counts can now be provided automatically.

The Coulter Corporation pioneered the development of monoclonal antibodies and flow cytometry. Wallace H. Coulter would often say there would come a day 'when we could go in and manipulate the cell', believing that monoclonal antibodies were the 'magic bullet' to cure cancer. He sold his company to Beckman Instruments in 1997 and, when he died in 1998, his estate founded the Wallace H. Coulter Foundation, Miami, FL.

In 2002, the foundation began its relationship with the ASH, providing the risk capital to establish the Clinical Research Training Institute, and the Highlights of ASH in Latin America and Asia. It also helped establish the ASH Lifetime Achievement Award. In 2009, the EHA launched its Outreach Program, to deliver education in haematology outside Europe. With the support of the Wallace H. Coulter Foundation, the EHA has organized educational activities in

Israel, Lebanon, Russia, Turkey, India, Kuwait, Ukraine, Estonia, and Armenia and hopes to include many other countries/regions in the future. In addition, the foundation helped to launch the Translational Research Training in Hematology, a joint effort between ASH and EHA.

Following the success of the Coulter Corporation, a number of other manufacturers entered the market. Sysmex introduced its first blood counter in 1963 and the first automated haematology system that combined cell analysis with slide-making and staining in 1988. They used fluorescence flow cytometry and cell counting methods to detect abnormal samples. However, although flow cytometry is now used for the white blood cell count and differential, for nucleated red blood cell detection, and reticulocyte counting, most manufacturers still use the Coulter principle of electrical impedance counting for parameters such as the red cell count.

Flow cytometry

Flow cytometry or immunophenotyping, as it is called in most haematology laboratories, changed the way in which we diagnose and classify leukaemias/ lymphomas and is also used routinely to diagnose some benign red cell disorders. Flow cytometry measures optical and fluorescence characteristics of single cells or parts of cells. In flow cytometry, cells are examined while they are flowing through a narrow flow channel. Firstly, a blood sample is diluted to a preset ratio and labelled with a proprietary fluorescence marker that binds specifically to nucleic acids. Then, the sample is illuminated by a semiconductor laser beam, which can separate the cells by using three different signals: forward-scattered light (forward scatter), side-scattered light (side scatter), and side-fluorescence light (side fluorescence). The intensity of the forward scatter indicates the cell volume. The side scatter provides information about the cell content, such as the presence of a nucleus and granules. The side fluorescence indicates the amount of DNA and RNA present in the cell. Emitted light is given off in all directions and collected via optics that direct the light to a series of filters and mirrors that isolate particular wavelength bands (colours). Cells with similar physical and chemical properties form a cluster in a graph known as a scattergram. At this point, a beam of monochromatic light, from a laser, intersects the cells. The light signals are detected by photomultiplier tubes and digitized for computer analysis.

Since their invention, flow cytometers have become small, easy to use, and cheap. Flow cytometric analysis is now an essential part of the classification of malignant haematological disorders and, as leukaemias and lymphomas often have subtle differences in their antigen profiles, they are ideally suited to analysis by flow cytometry. Diagnostic interpretations depend on a combination of antigen patterns and fluorescence intensity. Now analysers have at least three lasers (blue, red, and violet), whereas formerly they had a single blue (argon; 488 nm) laser which had a three-colour flow cytometry capability. The three-laser version allows the simultaneous detection of 8–10 different fluorochromes, as well as the two light scatter parameters. This trend is continuing, with the development of new fluorochromes and tandem dyes. Commonly used dyes include propidium iodide, phycoerythrin, and fluorescein.

Apart from the classification of malignant haematological disorders, measurement of CD4 numbers is used routinely to monitor HIV infection and response to treatment. CD34 numbers are also routinely assessed for in harvests for stem cell transplantation. In addition, flow cytometric analysis of erythrocytes has now virtually replaced the Ham's test in the diagnosis of paroxysmal nocturnal hemoglobinuria, and the Kleihauer–Betke test has been replaced by flow identification of erythrocytes that contain fetal haemoglobin. Assessment of platelet activation, qualitative platelet defects, and binding of immunoglobulin may also be measured by flow cytometry, although this approach has not yet reached the same level of acceptance as white cell or erythrocyte analysis. Nonetheless, the ability of flow cytometry to measure qualitative and quantitative abnormalities of all cell types and intracellular components (e.g. cell nuclei) has facilitated its transition from a research tool to a technique that is used in most clinical haematology laboratories.

Recombinant DNA technology and haematology

The large-scale synthesis of erythropoietin, a protein that regulates erythrocyte formation, is a good example of how recombinant DNA technology, which was developed in the late 1970s can be applied to haematology. In 1986 it was shown that recombinant human erythropoietin could correct the anaemia of renal failure (7), and in 1989 the FDA approved its use for the treatment of anaemia associated with renal failure. However, its use in the treatment of cancer/chemotherapy-related fatigue remains controversial.

Recombinant technology has also been used to manufacture other growth factors such as human G-CSF. The HIV crisis in haemophiliac patients stimulated the development of factor replacement therapy that did not originate from human plasma, and recombinant Factor VIII and recombinant Factor IX fulfil that remit. Nonetheless, although recombinant factors are often used in the treatment of newly diagnosed haemophiliacs, the cost of the factors is a major problem; thus, many countries still rely on plasma-derived concentrates. Moreover, with the widespread use of nucleic acid testing, the use of plasma-derived factor concentrates has never been safer.

Automated digital cell morphology

Initial attempts to automate differential white blood cell counting from a blood film in the 1970s and 1980s were hampered by the limitations of computers at that time. However, by the mid-1990s, computers had evolved considerably and were combined with artificial neural networks, which facilitated the development of automated digital cell morphology (ADCM) (8).

Probably everybody who reads this book has used a digital camera or owns a mobile telephone with a built-in digital camera. Digital imagery is probably the way forward for haematological morphology. ADCM analysers are now used in many haematology laboratories in Europe, although they are not yet as ubiquitous as mobile phones. Digital imaging was developed for the space programme in the United States, and the first digital images were created over 50 years ago. A digital image is a numeric representation of a two-dimensional image; each number represents the brightness and colour of a pixel, which is the smallest individual element in an image.

In the case of ADCM, the DM 9600, which is an ADCM analyser produced by CellaVision, for example, simplifies the process of performing differential white cell counts and creates an automated workflow for morphological cell analysis. Through the use of neural network technology, cells are automatically located on a stained peripheral blood film; images of the cells are then digitally captured, pre-classified, stored, and presented for confirmation. Remote review software makes it possible to access differential data from anywhere at any time, and the images may be kept indefinitely (Figure 11.3).

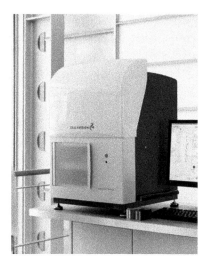

Fig. 11.3 The CellaVision DM 9600. The cell counter is attached to a display screen.

Reproduced with kind permission of CellaVision AB. Copyright © 2015 CellaVision AB, Lund, Sweden.

Staining

In order to visualize and differentiate blood cells, a method of staining had to be developed. The two names commonly associated with staining techniques are Paul Ehrlich (1854–1915) and Dimitri Leonidovich Romanowsky (1861–1921). In 1891, Romanowsky used methylene blue solution to detect malarial parasites in blood. Almost incidentally, he noticed that white blood cells were also brilliantly coloured by the solution. Romanowsky found that best staining was obtained when the methylene blue reagent was aged and had formed a surface film. For the next decade, many variations of Romanowsky's original stain were proposed by authorities such as Edward Jenner, Bernhard Nocht, William Boog Leishman, and others. In 1902 James Homer Wright and Gustav Giemsa both adapted Romanowsky formulations that are still popular throughout the world.

Many haematologists feel that the assessment of a patient is not complete until a well- prepared blood film is examined. Since the early 1980s, the International Council for Standardization in Haematology (ICSH) has published numerous guidelines/recommendations in laboratory haematology and staining of blood films and bone marrow aspirates (9–11). The ICSH was founded in 1963 and originally was closely associated with the European School of Haematology. Since 2007 the ICSH has been associated with the International Society for Laboratory Hematology. However, as we enter into the first quarter of the twenty-first century, many haematologists regret that examining a well-made blood film is becoming a 'dying art' among trainees.

The plastic bag

Changes in technology have affected all branches of haematology. In 1930 scientists working at Imperial Chemical Industries developed a new polymer they called polythene. This discovery was destined to change the commercial world and have a huge impact on blood transfusion medicine. The plastic bag became a reality but there were many technical problems to be overcome before use of the plastic bag for storing and transfusing blood became the norm.

Carl W. Walter (1905–92), a surgeon in the Peter Bent Brigham Hospital at Harvard Medical School in Boston designed the first polythene blood collection bag, which had an integrated donor line and a giving set. He and his colleague, William P. Murphy Jr, developed the flexible plastic bag, which was used for the first time during the Korean War (1950–3),[1] although, interestingly, in

---

[1] The Korean War also gave birth to the disposable, lightweight, airborne, liquefied gas expansion refrigerator for the transport of blood from the United States to Korea.

his article written in 1984, Walter never mentions Murphy (12, 13). In spite of its many advantages over the glass bottle in terms of weight, transportability, and rapid transfusion of blood under pressure, it took a number of decades before the plastic bag was widely used outside the United States.

Genetics and molecular medicine

Everybody agrees that the veritable explosion in genetic technology and molecular biology has profoundly altered medicine since the 1980s and deepened our understanding of the pathogenesis of diseases. These innovations have also given rise to novel approaches to therapy and hopefully will lead to curative therapy with little toxicity for the majority of malignant diseases. The fact that these novel techniques are mentioned throughout this book accentuates their ubiquitous nature throughout all aspects of the specialty. More details of genetics and gene therapy are contained in Chapter 9.

Fluorescence in situ hybridization

Fluorescence in situ hybridization, also known as FISH, was developed in 1980 (14) and since then has become widely used in haematology laboratories. FISH uses fluorescent probes which hybridize to complementary sequences. The resulting signals are examined under a fluorescent microscope. FISH probes allow multiple targets to be visualized simultaneously by using probes labelled with different fluorescent colours. FISH is routinely used to detect translocations such as t(9:22) and t(11:18), deletions such as 5q−, and Trisomy 7 and 8. Interphase and metaphase cells can be used in FISH. When used in clinical diagnoses, FISH is often used in parallel with cytogenetics and/or other molecular techniques (15).

PCR

Every haematologist knows the story of the genetic abnormality in the malignant cells of patients with chronic myeloid leukaemia, from the early observations of Peter Nowell and David Hungerford (although they were wrong when they thought that a small Chromosome 22, the so-called Philadelphia chromosome, was the genetic lesion in chronic myeloid leukaemia) (16, 17) to the demonstration of a reciprocal t(9:22) translocation by Janet Rowley (18). Subsequent understanding that the t(9:22) caused the malignant phenotype (19), leading to the development of tyrosine kinase inhibitors, made the story truly magic (20). Hundreds of thousands of people are now leading a normal life because of this development.

However if one asks, 'What is the most important technical development in haematology in the twentieth century', the technique of DNA amplification, otherwise known as PCR, must be a leading contender. Credit is given to Kary Mullis for improvements which he made in the PCR method when he worked for Cetus Corporation in California in 1983 (21). Although he shared the Nobel Prize for Chemistry, with Michael Smith in 1993, the original concept had been expounded 15 years earlier by Kjell Kleppe and Har Gobind Khorana in 1968 (22). Mullis, however, says he got the idea of using a pair of primers to bracket the desired DNA sequence and to copy it using DNA polymerase (a technique which would allow rapid amplification of a small strand of DNA) one night when driving with his girlfriend. The substitution of the heat-resistant DNA polymerase Taq, from *Thermus aquaticus*, by a colleague at Cetus made the technique affordable and amenable to automation. PCR made a huge impact on molecular biology and medicine, including haematology. Between 1985 and 2006 there was a huge increase in the number of publications about PCR (23) (Figure 11.4) and the technique has been used to detect leukaemia relapse (24), chimaerism following haematopoietic stem cell transplantation (25), and minimal residual disease (26). In haematology, PCR technology can be applied to cells obtained from bone marrow or peripheral blood.

Unlike FISH, PCR can only detect breakpoints covered by designated specific primers. Examples of the application of PCR include detection of *JAK2* V617F mutations, mutations in *FLT3*, *NPM1*, and *CEBPA* in acute myeloid leukaemia

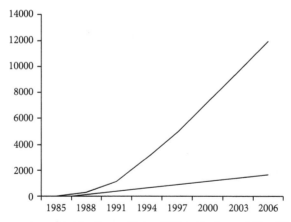

Fig. 11.4 The number of publications utilizing PCR, in the journal *Blood* (top line) and in the *New England Journal of Medicine* (bottom line), from 1985 to 2006.

with normal cytogenetics (27), and gene rearrangements, such as Ig heavy chain gene rearrangement in B-cell malignancies, and T-cell receptor gamma chain gene rearrangement in T-cell malignancies (28). Various extensions of PCR technology are widely used in haematology laboratories.

Haematopoietic stem cells: Where do we find them?

Traditionally, haematopoietic stem cells for transplantation were removed from the posterior iliac crest under general anaesthesia, and $1.0–2.0 \times 10^8$ mononuclear cells/kg of recipient body weight were subsequently transplanted. Although the lowest effective number of mononuclear cells is not known, graft rejection following allogeneic bone marrow-derived haematopoietic stem cell transplantation is not a significant issue. Stem cells had been demonstrated in the peripheral blood of mice in the early 1960s; but it was not until 1990 that Graham Molineux and colleagues demonstrated that successful haematopoietic stem cell transplantation could be carried out in mice given cells mobilized into blood following injection of recombinant granulocyte colony-stimulating factor (G-CSF) (29). Subsequently, William Bensinger and colleagues successfully transplanted patients with haematopoietic stem cells collected by continuous flow centrifuge in 1995 (30). The technique of collecting haematopoietic stem cells by continuous flow centrifuge using two peripheral veins has grown in popularity, and in 2013 the EBMT reported that most allogeneic haematopoietic stem cell transplantations used mobilized peripheral blood stem cells as a source of haematopoietic stem cells (31) (Figure 11.5). Donor safety is always a

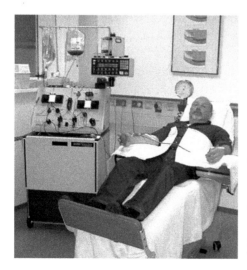

Fig. 11.5 A continuous flow centrifuge used to collect haematopoietic stem cells from the peripheral blood of a donor.

Reproduced with kind permission from the donor. Copyright © 2015 Shaun McCann.

concern but studies show that both procedures, marrow aspiration or collection of haematopoietic stem cells mobilized by G-CSF, seem to be safe and without significant long-term toxicity. A different approach to mobilizing stem cells is the use of the agent plerixafor. This drug inhibits the binding of CXCR4 on stem cells to CXCL12 on marrow stromal cells, thus releasing them into the blood. Most centres use haematopoietic stem cells mobilized with G-CSF and only use plerixafor in the autologous setting when G-CSF has not been successful.

The first successful cord blood transplant was carried out in 1988, and cord banks exist in many countries. A number of issues divide the transplant community. The expense of long-term cryopreservation and a sophisticated and reliable inventory system pose problems. The number of stem cells obtained from a single cord is relatively few, therefore a number of cords must be used for an adult recipient. The recent successes of haplo-identical haematopoietic stem cell transplantations may dampen enthusiasm for cord blood, as an EBMT study found a decline in the use of cord blood in 2013 in spite of an overall increase in transplant activity (31). The uptake of umbilical cord stem cells is still relatively slow, with the use of 30,000 units documented out of over half a million umbilical cord blood collections in storage (32). Efforts to expand the pool of stem cells by in vitro culture have not yet succeeded in overcoming the size disparity between adult recipients and cord blood volumes.

Technology and unrelated stem cell transplantation

Initial attempts at unrelated stem cell transplantation were hampered because inadequate methods of choosing donors led to increased rates of graft-versus-host disease, and graft rejection. Coupled with these problems, the majority of patients were referred for transplantation only when they had failed multiple alternative therapies and had suffered a lot of co-morbidity. The application of modern molecular-based tissue typing rather than serological methods, together with early referral, has yielded results for unrelated transplantation which are similar to those using fully matched sibling allogeneic haematopoietic stem cell transplantations.

What do we mean by 'fully' matched unrelated donors?

A number of PCR-based technologies are available, and this development has made HLA typing at the DNA level possible. These methods include the use of sequence-specific primers (PCR-SSPs), sequence-specific oligonucleotides (PCR-SSOs) and sequence-based typing. Sequencing, also known as Sanger sequencing, is the most direct and accurate method available. In this case, the DNA fragment is amplified by PCR and followed by base by base reading of each of the amplified DNA strands. The advantage of sequencing-based technology over PCR-SSP and PCR-SSO is its ability to analyse the entire amplified gene sequence, while the other methods can determine families of genetic polymorphism. This inability to resolve the family into specific tissue types is called ambiguity. Furthermore, even the power of sequencing-based technology has limitations, as ambiguity persists because this method cannot determine whether two polymorphisms, for example, are in 'cis' or in 'trans'. New or 'next-generation' sequencing methods are becoming available. Next-generation sequencing technology uses revolutionary chemistries that are different than those used in Sanger sequencing, enabling the resolution of ambiguity, sequencing of non-polymorphic regions, and sequencing in exponentially greater numbers (33). Using these techniques, it is possible to select fully matched donors or to allow 'permissive mis-matches'. Gottfried Fischer, the president of the European Federation for Immunogenetics pointed out the advantages of the new technology. He specifically mentioned next-generation sequencing and included as its advantages reduced cost (hopefully soon) and the generation of clonal sequences which relieve the issue of ambiguities. He also pointed out a potential 'downside' of this new technology, as high-throughput testing could replace or de-skill laboratory staff, so that small laboratories may lose the ability to detect the nuances involved in picking the most appropriate mismatched donor (34).

Various technologies have changed and improved the practice of haematology. Because of our ability to obtain blood cells so readily (via a simple venepuncture), haematology has been at the forefront of technological developments in medicine. The diagnosis of malignant and benign haematological disorders has become more exact because of the technological advances outlined, and our understanding of the pathogenesis of many diseases has been advanced as a direct result of the application of these technologies. However, it is important to stress that all technologies and 'tests' need to be cautiously interpreted, and a full history and physical examination should always be the first step in the investigation of patients.

References

1 Wintrobe M. Hematology, The Blossoming of a Science: A Story of Inspiration and Effort. Lea & Feibeger, Philadelphia, PA, 1985.

2 Bynum W. The History of Medicine: A Very Short Introduction. Oxford University Press, Oxford, 2008.

3 Minsky M. Memoir on inventing the confocal scanning microscope. Scanning **10** (4): 128–38. 1988.

4 Amos WB, White JG, Fordham M. Use of confocal imaging in the study of biological structures. Applied Optics **26** (16): 3239–43. 1987.

5 Thorburn AL. Alfred Francois Doneé, 1801–1878, discoverer of *Trichomonas vaginalis* and leukaemia. British Journal of Venereal Diseases **50** (5): 377–80. 1974.

6 Katayama I, Nagy GK, Balough K. Light microscopic identification of ribosome-lamella complexes in 'hairy cells' in leukemic reticuloendotheliosis. Cancer **32** (4): 843–6. 1973.

7 Eschbach JW, Egrie JC, Downing MR, Browne JK, Adamson JW. Correction of the anemia of end-stage renal disease with recombinant human erythropoietin. New England Journal of Medicine **316** (2): 73–8. 1987.

8 Hagner R, Wilson P. Automated digital morphology: Taking the 'manual' out of the 'manual differential', in KM Ward-Cook, CA Lehmann, LE Schoeff, RH Williams, eds, Clinical Diagnostic Technology. AACC Press, Washington, DC, 2006, Chapter 5.

9 Zanker V. ICSH reference methods for staining of blood and bone marrow films by azure B and eosinY (Romanowsky stain). British Journal of Haematology **57** (4): 704–10. 1984.

10 Scott DW, Den Ottlander GJ, Swirsky D, Pangalis GA, Vives Corrons JL, de Pasquale A, et al. Recommended procedures for the classification of acute leukemias. International Council for Standardization in Hematology (ICSH). Leukemia and Lymphoma **11** (1–2): 37–50. 1993.

11 Zini G, d'Onofrio G, Briggs C, Erber W, Jou JM, Lee SH, et al. ICSH recommendations for the identification, diagnostic value and quantitation of schistocytes. International Journal of Laboratory Hematology **34** (2): 107–16. 2011.

12 Walter CW. Invention and development of the plastic bag. Vox Sanguinis **47** (4): 318–24. 1984.

13 Barger AC. Some of Carl Walter's contributions to Harvard Medical School and Hospitals. American Journal of Surgery **148** (5): 578–80. 1984.

14 Bauman JG, Wiegant J, Borst P, van Duijn P. A new method for fluorescence microscopical localization of specific DNA sequences by in situ hybridization of fluorochrome labelled RNA. Experimental Cell Research **128** (2): 485–90. 1980.

15 Lam EPT, Chan CML, Tsui NBY, Au TCC, Wong KF, Wong HT, et al. Clinical applications of molecular technologies in hematology. Journal of Medical Diagnostic Methods **2**: 130.

16 Nowell PC, Hungerford DA. A minute chromosome in human chronic granulocytic leukemia. Science **132** (3438): 1479. 1960.

17 Nowell PC, Hungerford DA. Chromosome studies in human leukemia: Chronic granulocytic leukemia. Journal of the National Cancer Institute **27** (5): 1013. 1961.

18 Rowley JD. A new consistent chromosomal abnormality in chronic myelogenous leukemia identified by quinacrine fluorescence and Giemsa staining. Nature **243** (5405): 290. 1973.

19 Daley GQ, Van Eten RA, Baltimore D. Induction of chronic myeloid leukemia in mice by the p210bcr/abl gene of the Philadelphia chromosome. Science **247** (4944): 824–30. 1990.

20 Druker BJ, Talpaz M, Resta DJ, Peng B, Buchdunger E, Ford JM, et al. Efficacy and safety of a specific inhibitor of the BCR/ABL tyrosine kinase in chronic myeloid leukemia. New England Journal of Medicine **344** (14): 1031–7. 2001.

21 Mullis KB, Faloona FA. Specific synthesis of DNA in vitro via a polymerase-catalyzed chain reaction. Methods in Enzymology **155**: 335–50. 1987.

22 Kleppe K, Ohtsuka E, Kleppe R, Molineux I, Khorana HG. Studies on polynucleotides. XCVI. Repair replication of short synthetic DNAs as catalysed by DNA polymerases. Journal of Molecular Biology 56 (2): 341–61. 1971.

23 Brown PV. Personal communication. 2015.

24 Browne PV, Lawler M, O'Riordan J, Humphries P, McCann SR. Early detection of leukaemic relapse after bone marrow transplantation. Bone Marrow Transplantation 7 (2): 167–9. 1991.

25 Lawler M, McCann SR, Conneally E, Humphries P. Chimaerism following allogeneic bone marrow transplantation: Detection of residual host cells using the polymerase chain reaction. British Journal of Haematology 73 (2): 201–10. 1989.

26 Lawler M, Humphries P, McCann SR. Evaluation of mixed chimaerism by in vitro amplification of dinucleotide repeat sequences using the polymerase chain reaction. Blood 77 (11): 2504–14. 1991.

27 Zhang Q, Bai S, Vance GH. Molecular genetic tests for FLT3, NPM1, and CEBPA in acute myeloid leukemia. Methods in Molecular Biology 999: 105–21. 2013.

28 Evans PA, Pott CH, Groenen PJ, Salles G, Davi F, Berger F, et al. Significantly improved PCR-based clonality testing in B-cell malignancies by use of multiple immunoglobulin gene targets. Report of the BIOMED-2 Concerted Action BHM4-CT98–3936. Leukemia 21 (2): 207–14. 2007.

29 Molineux G, Pojda Z, Hampson IN, Lord BI, Dexter TM. Transplantation potential of peripheral blood stem cells induced by gralulocyte colony-stimulating factor. Blood 76 (10): 2153–8. 1990.

30 Bensinger WI, Weaver CH, Appelbaum FR, Rowley S, Demirer T, Sanders J, et al. Transplantation of allogeneic peripheral blood stem cells mobilized by recombinant human granulocyte colony-stimulating factor. Blood 85 (6): 1655–8. 1995.

31 Passweg JR, Baldomero H, Bader P, Bonini C, Cesaro S, Dreger P, et al. Hematopoietic SCT in Europe 2013: Recent trends in the use of alternative donors showing more haploidentical donors but fewer cord blood transplants. Bone Marrow Transplantation 50 (4): 476–82. 2015.

32 Ballen KK, Gluckman E, Broxmeyer HE. Umbilical cord blood transplantation: The first 25 years and beyone. Blood 122 (4): 491–8. 2013.

33 Sun Y, Xi Y (2013). The advanced HLA typing strategies for hematopoietic stem cell transplantation, in T Demirer. ed., Innovations in Stem Cell Transplantation. InTech, Rijeka, 2013. http://cdn.intechopen.com/pdfs-wm/42655.pdf.

34 Fischer G. European Federation for Immunogenetics Newsletter; 75: 2015.

Chapter 12

Combination chemotherapy

What price for curing haematological malignancies?

In a recent conversation, David Nathan told me that the major advances in haematology in his lifetime were automated cell counting, combination chemotherapy, and genetics (1). However, the claim that combination chemotherapy has been a major therapeutic advance is disputed by some who arguing that survival for most common cancers has not improved since the advent of chemotherapy (2).

It is certainly true that the survival of children with acute lymphoblastic leukaemia has improved and that the drug imatinib mesylate and its derivatives have changed the outcome for most patients with chronic myeloid leukaemia. Likewise, combination chemotherapy has greatly modified the prognosis for patients with Hodgkin lymphoma and some types of non-Hodgkin lymphoma. However, it must be said that the application of combination chemotherapy to common non-haematological cancers has not met with similar success.

The development of combination chemotherapy

Major wars have inadvertently had a profound effect on the development of haematology. Bone marrow transplantation developed from the Manhattan Project, which resulted in the atomic bomb in World War II, while chemotherapy began as an effort to develop chemical weapons during the same conflict. The bombing of the port of Bari by Germany during World War II resulted in the release of mustard gas into the atmosphere and the water, thereby demonstrating that the Allies were developing the potential for gas warfare. The existence of thousands of bombs of mustard gas in the US ship *John Harvey* was denied and covered up for a long time after the catastrophe.

Wintrobe, in his book *Haematology, The Blossoming of a Science* provides a detailed, if somewhat hagiographic, account of the early days of chemotherapy and the people who were the driving force behind its development (3). There is no doubt that Sidney Farber and Emil Frei III were very important in the early development of chemotherapy, but Wintrobe mentions many others, including David Galton, Jean Bernard, Rudolph Gross, Howard Earle Skipper, and James

F. Holland. We also owe recognition to a 'gentle man', Denis Parsons Burkitt (1911–93) (Figure 12.1). Burkitt was a medical graduate of Trinity College, Dublin, and, even though he had lost one eye as a child, his observations in Africa were seminal. In later years it was said that Burkitt went to Africa with one eye but saw more than most men with two eyes (4). Burkitt worked in Uganda and in 1948 was appointed as a surgical specialist to Mugalo Hospital, Kampala, and Honorary Teacher in Clinical Surgery, Makerere University College Medical School. His observations on a tumour of the jaw and abdomen in children are well known; this tumour, now called Burkitt lymphoma, was observed to be

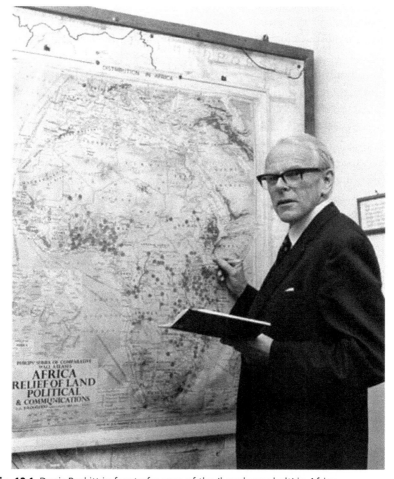

Fig. 12.1 Denis Burkitt in front of a map of the 'lymphoma belt' in Africa.

Reproduced by kind permission of Owen Patrick Smith. Copyright © 2015 Owen Patrick Smith.

dependent on altitude, temperature, and rainfall and was subsequently shown to be caused by Epstein–Barr virus reactivation by *Plasmodium falciparum*. Because Burkitt had no access to radiation, chemotherapy (then in its infancy) was the only option for treatment. Working with Joseph H. Burchenal (1912–2006), he obtained methotrexate gratis and was impressed with the tumour response. Burchenal and colleagues from the Memorial Sloan Kettering Cancer Centre developed the concept of combination chemotherapy in the 1950s and, for this innovation he, Burkitt, and 14 others were awarded the prestigious Lasker award in 1972 (5).

Combination chemotherapy, with or without radiation therapy, proved to be successful in the treatment of Hodgkin lymphoma, childhood acute lympho-blastic leukaemia, some subtypes of non-Hodgkin lymphoma, and acute mye-loid leukaemia. The use of combination chemotherapy for Hodgkin and non-Hodgkin lymphomas also provided very useful information on the short- and long-term toxicities of this treatment. The important milestones in the treatment of Hodgkin lymphoma are very well described by Sandra J. Horning from the Stanford Cancer Center (6); in the same article, she states that the disease serves as a paradigm for the effectiveness of combination chemotherapy with or without radiation in the treatment of cancer. More than 80% of patients with Hodgkin lymphoma are now cured, and current approaches, aided by fluorodeoxyglucose positron emission tomography (FDG-PET), are aimed at reducing toxicity. FDG-PET, usually accompanied by CT scanning in the same machine, provides a three-dimensional image of the tumour mass, and information on the metabolic activity (tumour activity) of the tissue under investigation. However, doctors need to be aware that PET-CT delivers substantial radiation to the patient (about 30 mSv) and that 6 PET-CTs will expose a patient to a radiation dose similar to the average A-bomb survivor (7). New treatments, such as monoclonal anti-CD30 linked to monomethyl auristatin E, are under investigation.

The treatment of childhood acute lymphoblastic leukaemia has been one of the great success stories of chemotherapy, with over 90% of patients now being cured and radiation therapy no longer being required. It has been clear for some time that acute lymphoblastic leukaemia is an acquired genetic disorder, and genetic analyses of acute lymphoblastic leukaemia cells facilitates stratification of treatment. The genetic abnormality and the early response to treatment help in choosing the appropriate therapy and, in some instances, reduce treatment with a view to limit toxicity. Current research therefore is directed at reducing therapy, limiting toxicity, especially long-term toxicity, and finding the best treatment for the 10% of children who relapse or fail to respond to initial treatment.

Acute myeloid leukaemia

The Medical Research Council, UK, has conducted many clinical trials of treatment for acute myeloid leukaemia and shown consistent improvement in outcome over time (8), particularly under the direction of Alan K. Burnett (Figures 12.2 and 12.3). However, a problem remains. Most patients with acute myeloid leukaemia are aged 60 years or more at presentation and do not qualify for most clinical trials. The outcome for such patients remains very poor.

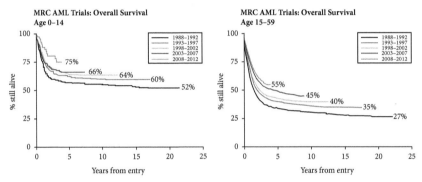

Fig. 12.2 A graph of overall survival rates from 1988 to 2012 for child (age 0–14; left panel) and young adult/adult (aged 15–59; right panel) patients with acute myeloid leukaemia, showing how outcomes have improved over time.

Reproduced by kind permission of Professor Alan K Burnett. Copyright © 2015 Alan K Burnett.

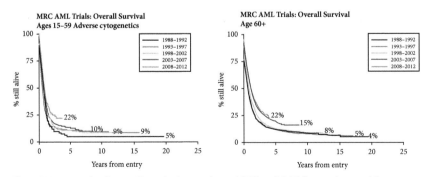

Fig. 12.3 A graph of overall survival rates from 1988 to 2012 for patients with acute myeloid leukaemia and who have adverse cytogenetics (left panel) or are >60 years old (right panel), showing how outcomes have improved over time.

Reproduced by kind permission of Professor Alan K Burnett. Copyright © 2015 Alan K Burnett.

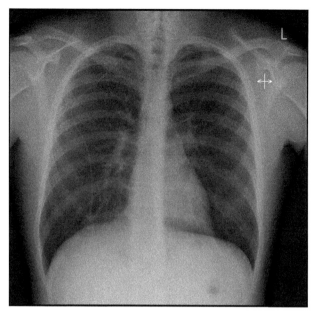

Fig. 12.4 A chest radiograph of a patient with a right atrial catheter in situ. Placing the tip of the catheter into the right atrium reduces the risk of thrombosis.

Reproduced with kind permission of Dr Ronan McDermott, St James' Hospital, Dublin. Copyright © 2015 Ronan McDermott.

Linking the anti-CD33 monoclonal antibody gemtuzumab to the cytotoxic agent calicheamicin (to form gemtuzumab ozogamicin (Mylotarg)) promised added efficacy but, unfortunately, is associated with marked toxicity. However, the strategy of combining monoclonal antibodies with cytotoxic agents will no doubt be the way forward when the problems of toxicity are overcome. Nonetheless, improvements in supportive care including venous access (right atrial catheters) (Figure 12.4), transfusion of platelet concentrates 'on demand', antibiotics and antifungal therapy, total parenetral nutrition, and radiological investigations and blood-based tests to detect infection have all undoubtedly contributed to the successful outcome for patients treated with combination chemotherapy.

Monoclonal antibodies

The idea that tumour cells could be eradicated if they expressed 'tumour-specific' antigens which could be identified has been around for a long time. The development of monoclonal antibodies in immortalized cell lines allowed

Richard Miller and colleagues to treat patients with non-Hodgkin lymphomas with so-called anti-idiotypic antibodies in 1981–82 (9). These were antibodies directed against tumour-specific antigens, notably, surface immunoglobulins which were expressed by tumour cells and were restricted to a single light-chain type and a particular variable region unique to each tumour. Although effective, this type of approach was technically difficult and time consuming and was eventually replaced by IDEC-C2B8 (rituximab), a chimeric anti-CD20 mono-clonal antibody.

The addition of monoclonal antibodies such as rituximab to chemotherapy has been very effective in the treatment of many patients with various forms of non-Hodgkin lymphoma, including diffuse large B-cell lymphoma, where it has significantly improved the outlook for patients with that disease. The com-bination of chemotherapy and anti-CD20 antibodies provides long-term disease-free survival in patients with follicular lymphoma and may lead to cure in some patients. Unfortunately, similar successes have not been experienced in the treatment of common solid cancers.

More recently the uses of monoclonal antibodies have widened to include immune-mediated diseases such as AIHA and immune thrombocytopenic pur-pura. Daan Dierickx and colleagues, in an excellent review, mention other hu-manized anti-CD20 antibodies which bind to epitopes other than the one that rituximab binds to and may thus be particularly useful in treating patients whose disease has become resistant to rituximab (10). The precise dosing and possible toxicity of monoclonal antibodies has yet to be determined but they certainly offer a completely new approach to the treatment of non-malignant immune haematological disorders. Thus, the success of chemotherapy has resulted in the development of new concepts of disease detection, and new treatments.

Minimal residual disease

The idea that small numbers of cells might remain after supposedly successful chemotherapy and lead to relapse of the primary disease led to the development of the concept of minimal residual disease in the early 1980s. The Rijswijk group, including Anton Hagenbeek and Dirk van Bekkum, developed the ter-minology by studying a rat model of acute myeloid leukaemia (7). Subsequently, Bob Löwenberg and Hagenbeek organized a number of seminars on minimal residual disease in leukaemia. In 1993 the concept of minimal residual disease was extended to indolent non-Hodgkin lymphoma in the autologous trans-plant setting by Armitage (11). Indolent forms of non-Hodgkin lymphoma lent themselves to the evaluation of minimal residual disease, as bone marrow in-volvement was particularly common in these disorders. Malcolm Brenner and colleagues then demonstrated that residual tumour cells contribute to relapsed disease (12).

Since these original observations, there has been an explosion of interest in the concept of minimal residual disease, since a sizeable fraction of patients achieving complete remission subsequently relapse and die from their disease (13). Quite a lot of effort has also been put into the possibility of 'purging' malignant cells from the inoculum before completion of the autograft procedure. The results remain controversial and may in part be explained by different 'purging' techniques and variables in the assay used to detect so-called minimal residual disease.

Assays used to determine minimal residual disease are PCR or flow-cytometrically based. Although PCR-based assays are more common, especially in lymphomas, both techniques have been compared in childhood acute lymphoblastic leukaemia and appear to be of equal sensitivity (14). PCR-based technology is used to detect tumour-specific translocations or antigen–receptor rearrangements. Detection of tumour-specific translocations is easier but not all patients have a measurable translocation in their tumour cells. Measurement of immunoglobulin heavy chain (IgH) and T-cell receptor genes is more complicated and may be unable to detect the malignant cells because of clonal evolution, especially in acute lymphoblastic leukaemia. However, detection of IgH gene rearrangements has been shown to be useful in 80% of lymphoma and myeloma patients, using PCR analyses giving specificity and sensitivity similar to results from translocation-based assays (15).

Should the detection of minimal residual disease dictate the patient's treatment?

The detection of residual disease by immunophenotyping or molecular assays will ultimately depend on sensitivity and reproducibility and the sample size. Robert Gale has been critical of using the detection of minimal residual disease, which he calls 'measurable residual disease', as a prognostic factor of disease in an individual patient, pointing out that a negative test for detection of minimal residual disease could simply be due to the small sample size (usually 5–10 ml). This possibility could explain why some patients in whom minimal residual disease cannot be detected will subsequently relapse (7). He also points out that many patients in whom minimal residual disease is detected after so-called remission induction and consolidation will not subsequently relapse. Mutations or translocations found in malignant cells may occasionally be found in normal individuals, and the malignant stem cell causing relapse may not show the same genotype or phenotype as the malignant clone.

He claims that we need randomized trials where patients who are positive for minimal residual disease are randomly assigned to placebo or conventional therapy.

In spite of these arguments, the detection of minimal residual disease has been used by many groups in deciding the necessity of further therapy in acute lymphoblastic leukaemia, chronic myeloid leukaemia, acute myeloid leukaemia, and lymphomas (16–18). David Grimwade and Sylvie Freeman echo in some way the views expressed by Gale, pointing out that there are a variety of methods for measuring minimal residual disease and stating that, until we have a standardized approach, we will not be able to include the measurement of minimal residual disease into clinical practice (16). However, the unravelling of the genetic and molecular abnormalities in diseases which a short time ago seemed to be homogenous has demonstrated that these malignancies are quite heterogeneous in nature and that the 'one-size-fits-all' approach to combination chemotherapy is being questioned. Similarly, the application of such an approach to minimal residual disease must be rigorously evaluated. However, Grimwade and Freeman say: 'With the range of platforms (in AML) [acute myeloid leukaemia] now available, there is considerable scope to realistically track treatment response in every patient' (16).

New technologies and the understanding of the genetic, epigenetic, and molecular abnormalities in haematological malignancies have facilitated the measurement of minimal amounts of disease and have changed our ideas about 'remission'. The question remains, can we eliminate all malignant cells with treatment and obtain a cure or can patients live for many years with minimal amounts of disease and a good quality of life?

Personalized medicine

The development of combination chemotherapy in the 1950s and the rapid growth of new technologies to evaluate molecular, genetic, and epigenetic changes in malignant cells have inexorably led to the idea of personalized medicine. The 'one-size-fits-all' philosophy which underpins combination chemotherapy may seem a little naive now, and it is clear that some patients will not respond to treatment while others, with ostensibly the same disease, will have a complete remission. A similar attitude can be taken to randomized clinical trials, for so long the 'gold standard' for evaluating the effects of drugs. Subgroup analyses may identify individuals with similar genetic profiles and whose disease shows an excellent response to treatment, a finding which may be lost if the group is evaluated as a whole. However, if these analyses are retrospective, they should be validated by prospective studies.

What do we mean by 'personalized medicine'? Surely all therapy is aimed at individuals and not diseases and is therefore 'personalized?' What current investigators, physicians, scientists mean by 'personalized medicine' is the tailoring of treatment to the molecular/genetic abnormalities present in tumour cells in order to effect cure with minimal toxicity. When associated with pharmacogenetics, it can also apply to non-malignant diseases. The term 'personalized medicine' may be misleading, as it does not mean that treatment will be 'personalized' for each individual; however, where groups of patients, usually with malignant disease, share genetic/molecular/epigenetic abnormalities, then treatment may be tailored for that group. As Hagenbeek says: 'One of the utmost advantages of personalized medicine is to prevent harm to the majority of patients' (19).

In 2010 Margaret Hamburg and Francis Collins (Commissioner of the FDA, and Director of the NIH, respectively) wrote a 'perspective' about personalized medicine in the *New England Journal of Medicine* (20); they said that, at that time, there was insufficient evidence to interest the pharmaceutical industry to invest in this type of research but that the NIH would promote it through programmes such as the Therapeutics for Rare and Neglected Diseases. They hoped that programmes such as that one would lead to discovery of molecular subtypes of common diseases and thus to new therapies. They stressed the importance of bio banks which could provide tissues for genomic evaluation. The authors issued words of caution, however. The success of personalized medicine would depend on accurate diagnostic tests and they pointed out that many of these tests have not been verified by independent investigators. They said that non-validated tests may miss the genetic abnormality which could advocate early intervention, or could overdiagnose the risk of malignancy. Their comparison, however, of personalized medicine to the creation of a national highway system in the United States is a rather reductive instrumentalist philosophical approach, common in that nation but not necessarily shared by the rest of the world.

A review in 2012 pointed out that, in haematology, although we know there are a number of polymorphisms in the genes that metabolize warfarin, it does not look as if genetic evaluation prior to beginning anticoagulation is a practical proposition in clinical practice (21). For example, clopidogrel requires activation by CYP2C19-dependent metabolism. Carriers of the *CYP2C19*2* allele will benefit from genetic screening in the setting of coronary artery stenting but not otherwise. Thus, personalized medicine would seem to be most suited to the treatment of malignant disease. However, acquired resistance, alterations in the genetic and epigenetic profile of the malignant cells, and the fact that leukaemic stem cells may not have the same profile as circulating malignant cells may limit the possibility of this approach to treatment of haematological malignancies. It is also important to remember that there may be considerable molecular heterogeneity between tumour cells in the same patient, making personalized medicine more difficult.

There is a large amount of interest in the concept of personalized medicine by the public, the media, and, to a lesser extent, the medical profession. There is a European Personalized Medicine Association and a Personalized Medicine Coalition, and the Third Astellas Innovation Debate (Astellas Pharma is a Japanese pharmaceutical company founded in 2005) called 'What the DNA and data revolution means for our health' was held in London, UK, in January 2015 (22). The debate, held in the Royal Institute London, UK, was moderated by the journalist Jonathan Dimbleby. The panellists were Baroness Helena Kennedy QC, Vice-President of the Patient's Association; Rolf A. Stahel, President of the European Society for Medical Oncology; Lionel Tarassenko, Head of Engineering, University of Oxford; and Leroy Hood, Director of the Institute of Systems Biology in Seattle, WA, and one of the ten scientists involved in the first sequencing of the genome of one individual. In this debate, George Freeman MP, who is Life Sciences Minister, said that the UK NHS would collect molecular/genetic data on 100,000 patients and match these with the patient's medical chart/notes. The information will then be shared with the pharmaceutical industry in an anonymized fashion. Whether this type of approach will yield useful results or not remains to be seen. Many people have grave doubts about the wisdom of agencies such as the NHS collecting large amounts of data on individuals, as people fear that the information might be used for nefarious purposes or might fall into the wrong hands. The public also fears that data can never be truly anonymized. Collecting genomic data on tumours is generally accepted but collecting data on the whole genome of patients is hotly disputed.

What was private is now public

Many interesting issues were raised in the Astellas debate but two, in particular, stand out. The attitude to privacy seems to be a generational one. Young people do not have the same regard for privacy as the over-60s, as witnessed by the posting of private information in social media. If genomic analyses are to become the 'norm', then it will require a complete overhaul of medical education and the education of thousands of genetic counsellors. As Tarassenko pointed out, the ability of a sophisticated and presumably highly educated audience to understand the mathematics of probability and concurrent probabilities is limited to about 5%. How then can we expect the public to understand these statistical concepts? Personalized medicine would also change the 'doctor–patient relationship', which we have believed in for over 2000 years. In response to a very interesting question posed by Jonathan Dimbleby, the audience were overwhelmingly opposed to the sequencing of an individual's genome at birth but a majority believed, at the same time, that such sequencing would eventually happen.

Private marketing of the human genome

23andMe is a privately held personal genomics and biotechnology company based in Mountain View, CA, with branches in many countries. It markets a saliva-based, direct-to-consumer personal genome test. In 2013 the FDA ordered 23andMe to discontinue marketing its personal genome service as the company had not obtained the legally required regulatory approval, resulting in concerns about the potential consequences of customers receiving inaccurate health results. The company, however, continues to sell a personal genome test without health-related results in the United States. It has been selling a product with both ancestry and health-related components in Canada since October 2014 and in the United Kingdom since December 2014. As mentioned above, most people's ability to understand probability and concurrent probabilities is very limited and there is a real danger of creating a large population of 'worried well'.

Although the public and the media have embraced the idea of personalized medicine, the medical profession does not seem to be as enthusiastic. Is this because doctors are afraid that patients will know more about their disease and genome than the doctor? Will the relationship between doctor and patient be altered by this type of information being made available to the patient? To a certain extent, this phenomenon may already be happening, given the amount of medical and genetic information available on the internet. The answers to these questions may become clear in the next decade, if and when personalized medicine becomes a reality for large numbers of patients.

Have we lost our way?

Of course, there have been many changes in medicine over the last 100 years, and life expectancy has dramatically increased in developed countries. The precise reasons for this increase are a little unclear, and life expectancy for patients with haemoglobinopathies still falls far short of the norm, even in developed, wealthy countries. Mass vaccination has undoubtedly helped, as has the provision of clean water. People do not often die from infectious diseases in developed countries, while diarrhoeal illnesses are still a major cause of mortality in children in developing countries.

We have made huge strides in understanding the pathogenesis of many diseases in haematology but this understanding has not always been converted into curative therapy. Likewise, apart from African Burkitt lymphoma, HTLV-III associated leukaemia, and gastric lymphoma, the aetiology of haematologic malignancies remains unknown. The molecular revolution has delivered very effective treatments for chronic myeloid leukaemia and HIV/AIDS and thus has had a huge impact on morbidity and mortality. However, these treatments remain expensive, and battles rage between pharmaceutical companies and the desire of doctors to provide inexpensive effective therapies. The media and some patients refer to haematologists as scientists. They are not. Yes, haematologists use scientific methods but they are primarily doctors, not scientists.

The main tenets of medicine, for thousands of years, have been careful history taking, a complete physical examination, and then appropriate investigations. As we have moved into the 'molecular' age we often hear criticism that doctors rarely shake hands, look into patients' eyes, or even take a history of the complaint. He/she looks at a computer and seldom engages the patient, who often finds this type of behaviour distasteful. I am not antediluvian, and patients, correctly, expect doctors to keep abreast of developments in their specialty. However, all the knowledge in the world about molecular pathogenesis is of little value without empathy and trust.

The growth of 'alternative medicine' surely makes it obvious that we have failed many patients. For those of us engaged in the training of medical students and young doctors, it is important to lead by example. No amount of sophisticated computer-based teaching can take the place of a well-given lecture from an expert who is a good communicator. Many of us have been inspired by a senior colleague but I have never come across a student or doctor who had been inspired by a computer!

The law of unintended consequences

The idea of unintended consequences dates to John Locke (1632–1704), who was a English philosopher and physician, and Adam Smith (1723–90), a Scottish philosopher; however, it was the sociologist Robert Merton who popularized the concept in the twentieth century. In his 1936 paper, 'The unanticipated consequences of purposive social action', Merton tried to apply a systematic analysis to the problem of unintended consequences of deliberate acts intended to cause social change. More recently, the law of unintended consequences is often used as an adage that an intervention in a complex system tends to create unanticipated and often undesirable outcomes. It is also commonly used as a warning against the hubristic belief that humans can fully control the world around them (23).

Is medicine a vocation?

The European Working Time Directive (EWTD) states that trainee doctors should not work longer than 48 hours, on average, per week (24). How long does it take to train a doctor or a specialist? Malcolm Gladwell in his book *Outliers: The Story of Success* examines the factors that contribute to high levels of success in business (25). Throughout the book, he mentions the 10,000 hours of practice that are required to become an expert. Whether you believe him or think he provides a simplistic approach to a complex problem, the EWTD makes it very difficult to train an 'expert'. The flaws in the EWTD were elegantly pointed out by Jonathan Osborne (Chairman of the Welsh Joint Consultants Committee, and Consultant ENT Surgeon) in 2006 (26). He claimed that, although the training in the United Kingdom had originally been based on the American resident system, the EWTD introduced a 'shift' culture, with the result that the trainee rarely sees his/her consultant to receive feedback. General surgical training has been reduced to 6,000 hours. He claimed that the EWTD is 'causing senior colleagues to worry about the standard of care they will receive in old age' (26).

The EWTD is implemented in various ways in different countries. According to a commission staff working paper, France and Ireland have not fully transposed the EWTD to doctors in training or have not fully implemented transposing measures (27). Consequently, the European Commission took Ireland to the European Court of Justice in March 2015 for failure to implement the EWTD, and Ireland may face a fine of €100 million. Such a penalty may be imposed on a country that is on its economic knees and where the health service is under severe financial strain. With manpower shortages in Germany, the opt-out appears to permit the extension of working time without compensatory rest. Such provisions are contained in public sector collective agreements for many hospitals. The EWTD (which is 176 pages long) concludes that there is a gap between the consensus reached by trade unions and that reached by employers. It also states that 11 member states claim that the EWTD has had a major negative impact. I could not find anywhere in the report any references to adequacy of training, or provision of care to patients.

Doctors may, of course, voluntarily remove themselves from the rulings of the EWTD. The rights of workers must be protected from unscrupulous employers but to limit doctors in training to specific hours diminishes the profession. Learning to be a doctor still relies on an apprenticeship model. As Aristotle said, 'One must learn by doing the thing, for though you think you know it, you have no certainty until you try'. The majority of experienced doctors with whom I have spoken believe that the EWTD is detrimental to training and patient care. This issue needs to be resolved.

References

1 **McCann S**. Interview with David Nathan on Views of the winner of the Wallace H. Coulter Award for Lifetime Achievement in Hematology Changes I have seen in hematology practice (audio): January 2012 [podcast]. http://www.multiwebcast.com/_ehapodcast/medias/17912_David_Nathan_audio.mp3, 2012.

2 **Bailar JC, Gornik HL**. Cancer undefeated. New England Journal of Medicine **336** (22): 1569–74. 1997.

3 **Wintrobe MW**. Hematology, The Blossoming of a Science: A Story of Inspiration and Effort. Lea & Febiger, Philadelphia, PA, 1985.

4 **Wright D**. Nailing Burkitt lymphoma. British Journal of Haematology **156** (6): 780–2. 2012.

5 **Clarkson BD, Foti M**. Joseph H. Burchenal: In memoriam. Cancer Research **66** (24): 12037–8. 2006.

6 **Horning SJ**. The cure of Hodgkin lymphoma, in 50 Years in Hematology: Research that Revolutionized Patient Care [brochure]. American Society of Hematology, Washington, DC, 2008.

7 **Gale RP**. Measurable residual disease (MRD): Much ado about nothing. Bone Marrow Transplantation **50** (2): 163–4. 2014.

8 **Burnett AK**. Treatment of acute myeloid leukemia: Are we making progress? ASH Education Program Book **2012** (1): 1–6. 2012.

9 **Miller RA, Maloney DG, Warnke R, Levy R**. Treatment of B-cell lymphoma with monoclonal anti-idiotype antibody. New England Journal of Medicine **306** (11): 517–22. 1982.

10 **Dierickx D, Delannoy A, Saja K, Verhoef G, Provan D**. Anti-CD20 monoclonal antibodies and their use in adult autoimmune haematological disorders. American Journal of Hematology **86** (3): 278–91. 2011.

11 **Armitage JO**. Bone marrow transplantation for indolent lymphomas. Seminars in Oncology **20** (5): 136–42. 1993.

12 **Brenner MK, Rill DR, Holladay MS, Ihle JN, Moen RC, Mirro J, et al**. Gene marking to trace origin of relapse after autologous bone marrow transplantation. Lancet **341** (8837): 85–90. 1993.

13 **Corradini P, Ladetto M, Pileri A, Tarella C**. Clinical relevance of minimal residual disease monitoring in non-Hodgkin's lymphomas: A critical reappraisal of molecular strategies. Leukemia **13** (11): 1691–5. 1999.

14 **Ryan J, Quinn F, Meunier A, Boublikova L, Crampe M, Tewari P, et al**. Minimal residual disease detection in childhood acute lymphoblastic leukaemia patients at multiple time-points reveals high levels of concordance between molecular and immunophenotypic approaches. British Journal of Haematology **144** (1): 107–15. 2009.

15 **Voena C, Ladetto M, Astolfi M, et al**. A novel nested-PCR strategy for the detection of rearranged immunoglobulin heavy-chain genes in B-cell tumours. Leukemia **11** (10): 1793–8. 1997.

16 **Grimwade D, Freeman SD**. Defining minimal residual disease in acute myeloid leukemia: Which platforms are ready for 'prime time'? Blood **124** (23): 3345–55. 2014.

17 **Yeung DT, Mauro MJ**. Prognostic significance of early molecular response in chronic myeloid leukemia patients treated with tyrosine kinase inhibitors. ASH Education Program Book **2014** (1): 240–43. 2014.

18 **Schrappe M.** Detection and management of minimal residual disease in acute lympho-blastic leukemia. ASH Education Program Book **2014** (1): 244–9. 2014.

19 **Anton Hagenbeek.** Personal communication. 2015.

20 **Hamburg MA, Collins FS.** The path to personalised medicine. New England Journal of Medicine **363** (4): 301–4. 2010.

21 **Gundurt-Remy U, Dimovski A, Gajović S.** Personalised medicine: Where do we stand? Pouring some water into wine: A realistic perspective. Croatian Medical Journal **53** (4): 314–20. 2012.

22 The Astellas Innovation Debate. The Astellas Innovation Debate 2015: iGenes: What the DNA and Data Revolutions Mean for Our Health. https://www.youtube.com/watch?v=2eaYgyRZQKo, 2015.

23 **Merton RK.** Social Structure and Science. University of Chicago Press, Chicago, IL, 1996.

24 European Parliament Council. European Working Time Directive. Directive No. 93/104/EC. 1993.

25 **Gladwell M.** Outliers: The Story of Success. Little, Brown and Company, New York, NY, 2008.

26 **Osborne J.** Modernising medical careers: An open letter to the Royal College Presidents. Journal of the Royal Society of Medicine **99** (2) 56–7. 2006.

27 EU Commission Staff Working Paper. Detailed report on the implementation by Member States of Directive 2003/88/EC concerning certain aspects of 'The Working Time Directive'.

Name Index

Subject Index